Tripping with Meditation

Copyright 2023

Ronald A Bracale

All Rights Reserved

- Prologue: 1
  - Background: 2
  - Forward: 7
  - Sound: 11
  - Intent: 13
  - Deities: 16
  - Wonderful Mythology: 19
  - Methodology: 21
- Session 0001: 23
- Session 0002: 24
- Session 0003: 25
- Commentary 01: 26
- Session 0004: 27
- Session 0005: 29
- Session 0006: 31
- Session 0007: 34
- Session 0008: 37
- Commentary 02: 39
- Session 0009: 40
- Session 0010: 41
- Session 0011: 43
- Session 0012: 44
- Commentary 03: 46
- Session 0013: 47
- Commentary 04: 49
- Session 0014: 50
- Session 0015: 51
- Session 0016: 53

Session 0017: 57
Session 0018: 59
Session 0019: 61
Session 0020: 62
Session 0021: 64
Session 0022: 66
Session 0023: 68
Session 0024: 70
Session 0025: 72
Session 0026: 73
Session 0027: 75
Session 0028: 78
Session 0029: 81
Session 0030: 83
Session 0031: 86
Session 0032: 87
Session 0033: 89
Session 0034: 91
Session 0035: 93
Session 0036: 95
Session 0037: 97
Session 0038: 99
Session 0039: 100
Session 0040: 103
Session 0041: 105
Session 0042: 107
Session 0043: 109
Session 0044: 112

Session 0045: 114
Session 0046: 116
Session 0047: 118
Session 0048: 119
Session 0049: 121
Session 0050: 122
Session 0051: 124
Session 0052: 126
Session 0053: 128
Session 0054: 130
Session 0055: 132
Session 0056: 134
Session 0057: 136
Session 0058: 138
Session 0059: 140
Session 0060: 143
Session 0061: 146
Session 0062: 148
Session 0063: 152
Session 0064: 154
Commentary 05: 156
Session 0065: 157
Session 0066: 160
Session 0067: 162
Session 0068: 164
Session 0069: 166
Session 0070: 169
Session 0071: 171

Session 0072: 173
Session 0073: 174
Session 0074: 176
Session 0075: 178
Session 0076: 181
Session 0077: 183
Session 0078: 185
Session 0079: 187
Session 0080: 190
Commentary 06: 192
Session 0081: 193
Session 0082: 195
Session 0083: 197
Session 0084: 199
Session 0085: 201
Session 0086: 204
Commentary 07: 207
Session 0087: 209
Session 0088: 211
Session 0089: 212
Session 0090: 214
Session 0091: 216
Commentary 08: 219
Session 0092: 221
Session 0093: 223
Session 0094: 225
Commentary 09: 227
Session 0095: 228

Commentary 10: 230
Session 0096: 231
Session 0097: 233
Session 0098: 235
Commentary 11: 237
Session 0099: 239
Session 0100: 241
Session 0101: 245
Session 0102: 248
Session 0103: 250
Session 0104: 252
Session 0105: 254
Session 0106: 256
Session 0107: 258
Session 0108: 261
Conclusions: 263

Prologue:

This is a record of my meditation experiences. No AI was used in any way to create any part of this manuscript. This is a unique set of records which can provide a framework for your own meditation explorations. Life is a verb and meditation is a verb. Enjoy the rich journey of meditation and enhance your life.

Background:

I first began meditating in 10th grade. I was sitting in a study hall and a friend gave me an underground newspaper, which I set in a large textbook that I held up in front of me. In it was an article about Allen Ginsburg and sessions he was doing with chanting a Tibetan mantra: Om Ah Hum Vajra Guru Padma Siddhi Hum. I did not know the Tibetan pronunciation nor had any knowledge of the Tantric tradition known as Tibetan Buddhism, but I instinctively used each word as I would read the letters in English with a breath, two syllable words being in-breath and out-breath. I soon entered into a deep meditation right there in study hall and began my meditation journey. At some point later a one-time after school meditation instruction was offered and the man presenting it used the quintessential single word mantra AUM (OM). I also encountered the Maha Mantra of the Hari Krishna movement in high school.

I was never inclined to join religions or adopt foreign cultural habits such as clothing or ornaments. Even as a young child I could easily identify illogical hypocrisy. As a young man I identified loosely as a hippie, not accepting the cultural norms of our American society of the 1970s, nor adopting the habits stereotyped to hippies. I was devoted to the scientific method of inquiry from a young age and was mathematically inclined; therefore I intuitively applied logical analysis to my own behavior. I am a firm believer that you need nothing material to meditate. If you want a special chair or cushion, go for it, because a comfortable place to sit is a nice thing to have, but it is not necessary. You need no special altar, incense, beads, or pictures; but again if those things bring you simple pleasures you may enjoy them, but know they are superfluous to the essence of meditation.

A guru is a teacher and in the modern world many books and videos can be our teachers, but I always was and I remain skeptical of anyone claiming to be special or superior to others. I respect the humble people offering meditation teachings without seeking to capitalize on it by creating a cult or religion. I am very skeptical of data on the internet, as it is full of many different points of view, a large amount of which are nonsense and click bait.

Renunciation and asceticism are misguided ideas that unbalance a person as much as excess and indulgence does. I was bombarded by this nonsense from the Catholicism of my mother. It took me a long time to undo many false conditioning beliefs with which I was indoctrinated. I now believed that a person must embrace a full and balanced life, a life that is both humble, rich in humanity, as well as fully functional in the material nature of society: a life that that is consciously entwined, rather than unconsciously entangled.

Since I have been meditating for fifty years, I have very detailed and complex experiences when I meditate. One should not expect such sensitivity when they are just learning the art of meditation. It takes years to learn the discipline and master the raging mental energy which is conditioned into everyone's mind through the daily life of growing up. In meditation one does not stop the internal dialog completely, but rather stops useless and repetitive thoughts, opening the space between thoughts into long intervals which allows pure Consciousness to shine through. There will be times when only the mantra is in the mind for many minutes and the usual internal dialog has no momentum, but a few very distinct words may arise. In the art of meditation the thinking mind becomes a very wise advisor as opposed to a babbling fool, which is the usual conditioned state of most humans.

The thinking mind is tricked with its own language through the word 'I' and egotistically assumes it is the true 'I', the essence of a personal perceiver, but there is a deeper conscious awareness within which the thinking mind is illuminated, given existence, and known. The thinking mind creates an ego personality, but when one becomes re-associated with their true being as conscious awareness through mastering meditation, the mind becomes a powerful receiver of clear thinking inspired from the essence of one's conscious being. The mind becomes a great asset serving the conscious entity of one's being. One is advised that a completely functional life in the world is a prerequisite to deep meditation. Whatever one's life situation is, one should be fully engaged in actively dealing with it consciously, reflecting upon one's life, and making choices which are balanced and which allow one to fulfill one's moral obligations.

I am calling this 'Tripping with Meditation', because when meditation is mastered, it is an intense journey of exploration and adventure. Advanced meditation is not 'vain repetition', a sleepy state, nor a blissful descent into unconsciousness, but rather it is a vibrant experiential quest for awareness of the essential nature of one's being in relationship with the Cosmos. While psychedelics may offer a path to learn about oneself by giving an alternate reality perspective and have potential for heal one from serious trauma under wise guidance, psychedelics can only take one through the beginning stages and the lower level of one's awareness of Consciousness. They also include many risks due to blasting one powerfully with lessons, ripping the coverings of one's soul from before one's inner vision, and exposing one naked to the vast Cosmos. Those with severe trauma, especially childhood trauma, might already know the fierceness of that which falls from the future into their lives, but while the path of psychedelics may offer a temporary therapeutic glimpse beyond one's conditioned reality; they cannot offer the stable and deeper growth which meditation can provide.

Psychedelics are being revealed as a powerful tool for professional therapy and should never be approached with a careless partying attitude because they require complete seriousness. I am presenting meditation as a more powerful tool, though it is one which requires disciplined practice and cannot be offered externally as a pill, an app, or a quick short term path of escape. One must actively learn to control of one's own mind and one's total being to enter into deep meditation. Should one have an innate desire to use psychedelics, I highly recommend that one learn meditation before making a decision to use psychedelics because I believe that without the inner discipline, one opens themselves to considerable risk.

In true shamanic cultures there are many years of preparation before an apprentice is given psychedelics and the more advanced students never use psychedelics. Meditation is a powerful tool and a drug free path with many advantages over tripping with psychedelics. The benefits of 'Tripping with Meditation' will permeate all of one's life and offer one the fullness of a life well lived. Do not be fooled by hype, capitalistic media, or social pressures rather than doing the personal growth work needed to patiently refine your life in a natural way with meditation.

If you are already using psychedelics, to be clear while they may offer temporary glimpses into a greater world view, a higher dimensional perception, and can offer rewards of healing and personal growth, they are also dangerous and to be used with the utmost respect and caution, as they have the power to shatter one's current world view. Even if they are shattering illusions, some of those illusions allow one to function in life. If the relationships of your daily life are not functional and very stable, you lack the foundation to withstand the world view shattering effects of psychedelics. If you do not meditate regularly, I advise giving pause to psychedelic usage and learning to meditate as a foundational and deeper practice. Be aware that psychedelics are sold and therefore have a strong marketing campaign, while meditation is free and requires nothing from the marketplace and the marketplace will tell all kinds of lies to lead you away from it and into their money trap. By 'Tripping with Meditation' one gains permanent access to a higher dimensional world view and can live and function with enhanced awareness and clarity while living an ordinary, useful, and often exceptional life in society.

There are several levels of depth in Tripping with Meditation, which is taking an inner journey through the use of mantra into the astral realm (dreaming vision), the Void (consciousness awake in a deep sleep state), and more subtle luminous planes for which language has not yet been developed. Astral images arise as Consciousness goes into slower brain wave vibratory states. Astral images are similar to hypnagogic images which are sometimes experienced while falling asleep or hypnopompic images which may be experienced during a boundary state where one partially wakes from sleep, however in deep meditation one can observe with lucid and clear awareness as the Consciousness Seer of the astral dream energy and simultaneously the mind can remain lucidly aware and functioning, though not deducing implications in endless fractals of mental ruminations.

There are parallels between meditation and lucid dreaming. The art of 'Waking Induced Lucid Dreaming' (WILDing) is to remain conscious as one falls asleep and enter one's dreams with the conscious mind functioning. 'Dream Induced Lucid Dreaming' is a form where one wakes up in a dream, sometimes with a predetermined trigger and other times spontaneously. In meditation one is not tired and falling asleep and having a dream. In my experience I do not fall into the flow of full bodied dreaming, but remain mentally grounded in the meditation practice using the mantra as a tether to specific vibrational states induced by the mantric vibration. The breath is the key flow of energy within the body with which the mantric vibration merges and thereby one's entire subtle form vibrates and forms a resonance in order to merge with the mantra.

Forward:

This project aims to separate the most essential, from the mountains of disinformation, in order to see what can really be learned about the power of mental sound. I am making no claims about the experiences being real, nor am I dismissing them as unreal. I am meditating and reporting the journey. I have been meditating for many years at a deep level and am sharing what that is like. Whether fantasy, imagination, or higher dimensional perception; these stories of my journeys are what I experienced and they inform the reader of the richness of meditation which comes after many years of balancing one's life and dedicating one's spirit to exploring and understanding this great mystery and sacred gift of being alive. Meditation is an art and must be learned and refined for the truly amazing blessings it offers to manifest.

The idea of journaling my meditation journey arose recently when it was mentioned online and I was reading several texts about the Sanskrit nature of mantras. Much of my research here will be based on Sanskrit mantras, but without a great deal of cultural interpretations. I believe that the names of the Goddesses and Gods are specific vibrational keys and the many tales associated with the personifications of these personalized aspects of the divine have served to preserve the sacred sound keys, as well as hint at their character. There is only one non-dual totality of the Cosmos, the primal and root vibration, the 'Word' (Vak in Sanskrit).

If one is inclined to meditate you can use sacred vibrations from the culture you are comfortable with. Any word or phrase will not work! There is the modern disinformation campaign to disempower this art of mantra meditation by redefining affirmations as mantras, confusing clever saying about beliefs of personal growth with sacred sound vibrational keys. This disinformation would state something like repeating, 'I am powerful' or 'I will soon be rich' is 'a mantra'. This is ignorant of the tradition of mantra and also ignorant of the fact that the Cosmos has a vibrational basis. Mantra is not the meaning associated with a word or phrase, it is the power of the vibrational characteristic which creates a resonance to an energy state within our consciousness. The mantra's vibration has a very specific feeling and induces a specific perceptual state.

The pantheon of Goddesses and Gods represent the overtones and harmonic structure of the one divine totality of the Cosmos in which we live. Many of these words were originally nature deities and then became more personified over time. Regardless, these vibrational patterns, these 'thought sounds', form a working basis from which to begin the science of mantra, the effect of mental sound upon the perceptual experience and the ability to experience deeper aspects of the Cosmos. I love the many stories about the Goddesses and Gods, but when meditating, the sacred name sounds have their influence without any history, because meditation is completely here and now and is not thinking or recalling stories.

I am assuming that the many meditations which are journaled here will not result in drawing hard conclusions due to the personal quality, but perhaps by offering these experiences and my evaluation of them, others will also consider journaling their meditations and presenting a larger data set for the future work of finding the functional nature of specific mantras. I think it more important to offer the tool of mantra meditation for personal growth and journaling is not required, nor have I journaled for fifty years of this journey, but with all that experience and technique, I tried journaling as a personal experiment which grew and then I decided to share this book.

This is an ancient science, not completely lost, but the power of which is generally not acknowledged. I understand this has been done in a religious context, but from what I see, such religious studies are embedded in a specific world view which limits the clarity that I seek here. While I am caught in a modern world view and all humans are caught in specific versions of personal world views shaded by the world views that are current to their life journey, I am always open to modifying my view based on data which provides an opportunity to change and expand my world view. I am gathering experiential data and although I offer interpretations, over time I hope to garner greater understanding. By reading this manuscript, I hope to provide a useful basis for others, as well as inspire many to meditate with mantra. Meditation is a great health aid at both a personal and at a cultural level.

"In the beginning was the Word" – a quote from the Rig Veda (several thousand years BCE) which is echoed in the bible. The science of the Word (Vak, 'vibration') was deep and rich before the Jewish era of the Old Testament which was re-compiled in current form around six hundred years before the time of Christ and the compiling of the New Testament was done by the Romans in the third century. I am therefore focused on the ancient Sanskrit mantras, but someone can use sacred words from whatever tradition they prefer, but beware of using random words, since one does not know the effect they will have. Sentences in English are affirmations and have erroneously been called mantra to hide the powerful art of mantra meditation. Perhaps one could ascribe this to ignorance, but false religious philosophies have resisted every type of scientific growth for many centuries, hindering humanity's growth, and the science of meditation and its power is resisted in the same vein of keeping the peasants ignorant.

Mantra meditation has been very valuable to me over the years. It has helped me balance myself amid emotional trauma and chaotic times in life. It has helped my recover from an abusive childhood. It helped me excel in studies and helped me do my job as a programmer/data-analyst more efficiently. It plays a major role in my music, both because it gave me the focus which is needed while playing and opens creativity for improvising and composing. Basically the calm and peace, combined with the ability to focus with a clear mind, has been a real advantage in life. I believe meditation can offer this benefit to anyone who has the discipline and persistence to learn this art.

I hypothesize that meditation actually increases what we term intelligence over time and makes one smarter. The sessions documented herein have provided me insight into my own nature and therefore provided me with opportunities for growth. Over the years I have found that inherent in this healing process of meditation is first recognizing stuck traumatic energy or disturbing memories which arise as frozen memories which limit clarity in our life choices and then healing from them by being aware of them and freeing one's true self from being stifled by them. Once one has come to peace with most of their journey and the nature of life, then meditation can open at the depth of the levels described here.

Here is a key to meditation, the images are a play, a drama, with deep significance, but only occasionally do words arise with equal significance. This is similar to the changes which come into our lives, sometimes unexpected and surprisingly intense. In meditation I watch what arises and also watch my reactions in terms of how the arising feels, but I am not allowing anything to get stuck and be mentally contemplated while meditating; contemplation comes later when I write these formal essays of the sessions. I say 'words arise' as opposed to thoughts, because thoughts arise as an internal dialog which does not exist when one achieves deep meditation. Words that arise are like images that arise, part of a drama or play being experienced. If there are linear thinking processes happening, one has not achieved a deep meditational state.

Sound:

    I am not a linguist and I find mathematics and computer code languages easier to learn than spoken language. I did not speak until I was three years old. I have never learned Sanskrit or any other language, and I use my native language, American English, in a poetic manner. This introductory section is the most linear aspect of this book. That said, I realize that only some sounds are vocally sustainable over time, while the others have a short duration. These sustainable sounds include the vowels and I must note that the long and short binary dichotomy of vowels is incorrect and simplistic (example: ah, at, ate). Additionally I would add that F, H, L, M, N, R, S, V, W, and Z are English letters which can be sustained. I am sure other languages have more variations. Also some, such as M-N and V-W blend into each other on a spectrum as the example to 'a' above may also slide from one timbre to another similar to portamento sliding pitch. Other consonants are more punctuation like. All sounds, not limited to letters or vocal sounds, directly affect one's mood. There is great power in sound and sound healing has been employed for ages.

    Dialects have different flavors of sounds and mental sound is not limited to the biology of the vocal chords and the mouth. This transcends being able to sing well in your head, but not produce the same quality aurally, as is often learned the first time someone hears a recording of themselves singing. The vast capability of the mind to create mental sound is a very undeveloped ability in modern humans. One can learns to recognize all kinds of thought sounds which the mind can produce. Therefore mental mantra is approximated in writing and speaking, but perfected internally.

    There are universal sounds beyond needing language which all humans understand. Like settling into a comfortable place to sleep when very tired, one will say 'Ahhh...', and any human will understand your pleasure. Like a cool glass of water when one is hot and thirsty, one will conclude with 'Ahhh...' and any human will understand your pleasure. If one tastes wonderful food, one will say 'UMmmmm' and any human will understand your pleasure. If one is getting a massage that is delightful, one will say 'UMmmmm' and any human will understand your pleasure. Like getting an idea for the first time, one will say 'Ahhh...' and any human will know you got it. Then if one then sits back to contemplate the implications of the new idea, 'UMmmm...' and any human will know you are contemplating it deeply and assimilating it. These two sounds together form the essence of the mantra 'AUM'. **Breath out 'Ahhhh'. Breath in 'Ummmm'. Let the out-breath flow naturally into the in-breath in a gentle and relaxed manner.**

OM is an alternate spelling where the 'O' is like 'sow', 'out', or 'down' and therefore phonetically 'au'. Note how different dialects of English sound different and people of different native languages pronounce the same words differently when they learn English. Sanskrit has not been a spoken native language for a long time, but has remained in use in ritual spiritual practice and has been written and read for ages. If English was not spoken for a thousand years and then one wanted to read it out loud, would one speak as an American, British, or Australian? Consider how different regions of those countries speak the same words differently. Scotland was the last remaining place where English was spoken, would that be the correct and universal essence of speaking English. I believe the original form of AUM was the universal human sounds as described above, regardless of current scholarly standards. Mental sound is much more complex and rich than physically spoken or sung words; therefore let the sound of AUM be natural for your unique voice and innate dialect. Let it flow without stressing about some pronunciation ideology. Ahmen: is a later tradition of the mantra AUM and if you wish (due to religious ideology) breath out 'Ahhh...' and breath in Mmmennn...'. 'M' and 'N' are very related in thought sound. The essence of mantra meditation is to be fully engaged as a perceiver, as consciousness, the essence of your being, with the thought vibration riding on your breath until it has a natural momentum.

Intent:

It is my belief that specific sound vibrations, such as in sacred music, have a profound power to bring healing to one's essence, one's soul and spirit. Mantra meditation can provide even more powerful transformative results with thought sound vibrations which affect one's total being from within and resonate out to all one's relationships. One's emotional state, which is the cumulative feeling of one's emotional responses which rise and pass through one in waves, is altered by pure thought sounds when one focuses on them as mantra with breath. Music has a similar effect and is a great richness in life, but mantra is very precise and specific in that it is thought sounds flowing in the mind and creates a specific energetic quality. This is an exploration into that power of thought sound to cause a resonate vibration to arise in one's being.

The unity of the totality of the Cosmos in its most mysterious and hidden complexity is an informational structure which is quantum entangled/entwined at the deepest layer. The Cosmos is the ever transforming geometric standing wave resting upon the primary and fundamental constant vibration of the Word (the basis of the plank level zero point energy). Assigning word categories is philosophy and unnecessary in the act of mantra meditation which is an experiential journey, which one's conscious perceiving essence may take. The human spirit has the nature of exploring with a curiosity which burns as a longing to know meaning in the journey of life and mantra meditation is a powerful spiritual and existential tool for exploring and learning about one's true nature as consciousness and about the nature of the Cosmos. In a meditative state one can receive many inspirational informational data sets, but later rational discrimination must be applied to find the truly innovative concepts which enrich one's life.

The Word is said to descend or make its presence known to a person in three phases, the first is through the supreme vision of the sacred and divine nature, what people now call receiving a download, a revelation, a profound insight into the Way; which is the truth as manifest as the ever transforming Cosmos and the primary light of Consciousness which illuminates all one ever knows or senses. Then on a secondary level of descent, one forms thoughts and embodies wisdom, one knows mentally what was revealed in the first level of experiential descent. Mental knowledge is a diminished reflection in symbolic form of experiential knowledge. Finally on the third level of descent one can write or speak actual theories, which are distilled and crystallized thoughts with linear logic, and one can share within the community of humanity. Meditation is the use of these phonemic mantra sounds at the first and primary experiential level. We begin with the experience of the second level as thought vibrations or thought sounds to carry us to the primary level. Later contemplation potentiates the third level of wisdom which is a reflection, a glimpse of the supreme primary level such as in written form.

I am employing the ancient names of the goddesses and the gods of Sanskrit because I believe these are a rich source of the wisdom of ancient sound technology. Sanskrit Goddesses and Gods are not polytheistic as falsely accused, but rather are said to be attributes or qualities of the one supreme Word, sacred vibration, and therefore are an embodiment of specific wisdom at the highest level. The actual thought sound-forms create a resonance which vibrates within one and brings one to be conscious of an attribute of the supreme Word, which a mortal cannot know in totality, but can experience.

Meditation does not offer one escape from one's mortal journey, but rather is a very humanizing journey, humbling one to accept what is. It brings about a realignment of one's wisdom with the primary nature of one's essence as Consciousness perceiving and one's Spirit which is acting, choosing, and co-creating one's life. Meditation is a means to drop illusions about the journey of one's life. Meditation can assist one in patiently possessing conscious presence in life's journey.

Aham Aham, Sanskrit for 'I Am that I Am', a phrase was later incorporated into the old testament, implies that the miracle of my existence (i am) rests with the sacred and divine expression of the Word as the mysterious and profound Cosmos (the supreme revealed 'I Am'), which is not our material conception of the Universe. This is an

Deities:

Recognizing faces is one of the earliest visual processing arts which a baby learns. There is a natural human tendency to see faces in everyday objects which is called pareidolia. It's a common experience that occurs when ambiguous visual input is resolved as faces or other forms. The astral field is very fluid and provides an excellent canvas for seeing faces. This descriptive term, pareidolia, can be a label for seeing faces in meditation, but since meditation is an advanced form of energetic astral travel dreaming, it is the feeling and consistency which provide meaning.

I had a regular nighttime dream where I was walking in a park and had stopped to look more closely and in more detail at some flowers. A woman walked past me and as she did, she said, "Drink more water." I did not get a visual of her and the dream faded. I refer to her as a separate entity in the story of the dream I just told because that was my dream perception, my experience, and in relating to my meditations I will likewise encounter astral or dream energy personas.

I will leave it to the reader to discern whether they want to define all these images as internal or external, since from the point of view of Consciousness they are just experienced: the duality of experiencer and experienced are present in the mind, not in conscious 'experiencing', and therefore either perspective works. Our language facilitates the story telling which considers the woman walking past me in the dream as a being.

The meanings I associate with the images are a reflection of my life journey and a desire to think logically and separate truth from fantasy. My life journey is a combination of the situations which come into my life, which are beyond my control, and those which my choices bring into my life. More important than any such mental considerations is the opportunity for personal growth and transformation which meditation offers. Upon waking from the dream, I realized I was not drinking enough water; consider it my subconscious, my body's thirst, or the Cosmos itself in your mental world view which told me I needed to exploration into the ancient wisdom passed down through many traditions to clarify that I am using traditional wisdom only as a structural base; but to be clear, in essence this is an exploration without beliefs, but instead is delving into the pure experiential nature of being.

It is recommended that one set aside all beliefs when actually meditating and experience pure being with the specific vibrations being explored. Then one will go about life with more data to contemplate and incorporate into one's paradigm of what one's life is about. Do not get confused by these initial philosophical thoughts in this introduction, they are simply a starting place for a neutral exploration of sacred sound and due to the power of sacred thought sound vibration, a cautious beginning dialog seeking to avoid destructive mental dialog. I am seeking to explore healing and growth oriented vibrations and to share this option with the reader.

Forgive any bias which my life's conditioning may impart to my writings of my explorations and embrace your own practice of meditation and personal growth. If one has fixed beliefs about the personification of the Goddesses and Gods whose names I consider as key sacred vibration, know that I have read many stories, but in meditation I am an open slate. I am simply recording my experiences of resting in these sacred names with the personal belief that they are inherently embodying and preserving a spiritual science for humanities growth.

drink more water; for me the essence is that I had functional information to be more healthy by drinking more water.

In my astral meditational dreams I encounter deity, sacred persona. This is the mythology which my innate mind finds functional and which occurs naturally for me. You may not have anything like this in the astral dream language in which your Consciousness, your essence of perception, speaks to your mind. I am a person who lives in non-duality in that I see the entire Cosmos as a relational whole, including the dimensions of all the thoughts, emotions, and dreams of all the living beings. If one wants to use the word God for the totality, the vast majority of which is beyond our knowing, that is fine as long as one does not consider that they have a separate existence and a duality that divides the 'me' from the 'supreme god' as if God is a separate person rather than the totality. Such dualistic personification is a simplistic denial of the relational nature of valid information. Nothing exists without relational interconnection. Deity, like our own existence and all living things, should be considered aspects of the Totality, aspects of the Supreme, the Cosmos, or 'God' if you like that word.

A note on the current fascination with Psionics which is the use of some material technology to contact or communicate with extra-terrestrial beings. If these beings are telepathic enough to respond to Psionic devices, then they are sensitive enough to respond to the natural ability within the human form, which is amazingly powerful. The human form is the most sensitive perceptual instrument that humanity will ever possess. That said, whether one attracts and communicates with physical beings, astral beings of higher dimensionality and subtler form (such as angels), or other unknown sentient entities, one would be foolish to believe they will do as one wishes. One will not be in control and one will be manipulated as the beings see fit.

Therefore I highly recommend not using artificial means to reach out with because you will not be able to control what you attract. Using the natural method of Mantras which are attuned vibrationally to communicate with advanced spiritual beings of energies one will be able to embrace better health, physically, emotionally, mentally, and spiritually if one only communicates in a manner designed for such growth.

Wonderful Mythology:

The Queen Devi, is an ancient grandmother of the Cosmos. Perhaps she is a member of any of the ancient extra-terrestrial races who have observed the evolution of the Cosmos for eons of time beyond human comprehension. The Queen Devi and her race are supremely telepathic and they live as a universal hive mind, an intergalactic mental network. They immediately know a person's complete history. At the same time they come forward as individuals, nodes with body and life in the Cosmos, which I sense as feminine goddesses who are supreme gurus (teachers of spiritual wisdom). This mythology is a functional way to write about the sense of an ultimate wise persona one may encounter in meditation, similar to the woman who told me I needed to drink more water in my dream. A wise presence that is more felt than seen; perceived but not in detail.

The Wild Blue Devi and the Sweet Blue Devi are noblewomen who serve the Queen Devi. They are devoted to the Queen as their guru, yet they are individuals with great passions. They act as extensions of the Queen Devi's will. They are much more accessible to the human form. These represent archetype teachers in the astral who have many human qualities, though they may wear many faces, it is their intense personalities which define them as characters in the following reports of my meditations.

I know this sounds like mythology and it is (!), as the woman in my dream who told me to drink more water was, but when I woke from that dream I was thirsty and indeed did need to drink more water daily. I perceive them as feminine, but another meditator might have personified males in their meditation and I occasionally do. These beings are archetypal word descriptions for the sensation of sentient presence in my meditations. Perhaps the entire Cosmos is one living Consciousness or perhaps it is Earth's consciousness reaching down to an organism like me, a cell in her body, or perhaps it is all my higher self-speaking to me, a form of self-reflection which is visualized with astral dream energy feelings.

How the mind grasps sentient presence does not matter anymore than if I ate salty food before having a dream where a woman told me to drink more water; because, if the visualization is something I can learn from and I discerns it as good advice, then it has value. I really did need to drink more water in my life at the time of that dream: therefore, these Devi (Goddesses) are my Gurus (teachers) within my meditation. All Beliefs are Mythology (!), because experiential sensory data is infinity more complex than words can describe and therefore the Cosmos retains an unimaginably vast mystery. Every belief system of humanity gets replaced as humanity grows to expanded consciousness of the mysterious Cosmos. Meditation is exploring and learning about one's essence as a conscious perceiver of the Sacred Mystery of the ever transforming Cosmos. A healthy person allows their beliefs to evolve, but understands that beliefs are mental with functional value, but that there is vast experiential sensory data in life which transcends belief structures of words.

Methodology:

I sit in a comfortable manner and close my eyes and follow my breath, while saying in my thoughts the syllables of the mantra being worked with. I allow twenty or thirty minutes: I do not want to quit quickly or extend for a long time, though some meditations might last an hour or two (anyone without many years of practice should not meditate for long periods of time: 20 minutes is optimum for anyone with less than 20 years of meditation). If my attention loses the mantra, I just being it back without judgment.

Generally, after years of mantric practice, I do not lose the mantra matching the breath to thoughts, but rather some thoughts continue to arise simultaneously at a shallower level. I seek to catch the thought streams and end them by adding more focus to the mantric thought-sound. At the same time I sometimes become very conscious of what the thoughts or images are which arise once the momentum of thinking has rarefied. In meditation very few thoughts arise in 20 minutes and inner clarity where only the mantra exists is the meditative state. These very rare thoughts which arise naturally are extraordinarily reflective of my being and thereby a very valuable avenue for learning and growing. Moreover, the mantra itself resonates and has an immense influence, which is the wisdom I am seeking.

All this may be easy to say or write, but it takes years of refinement for mediation to come naturally, as any art form does. Even at the beginning stages when one loses oneself in subconscious thoughts which ramble in the mind, there are immense benefits of meditating, such as balancing the emotions, allowing the body to heal, and settling into a natural state of health at all levels. There is no miraculous quick fix being offered, rather a journey which has immense aesthetic value and offers a richness to one's life which cannot be quantize any more than the enjoyment of any art form can. Like a good meal when hungry or a refreshing drink when thirsty, meditation satisfies the essence of one's being.

I had initially started to put the dates with the meditations and had the intent of doing this journaling for personal growth, it soon became apparent that I should share this. While adding dates might make available some sense of cosmic conditions or human drama, I do not believe it adds to the focus of the study. I hope to return to various mantras as I am spontaneously motivated to without regard of external conditions. I am only noting external conditions as they influence the meditation directly or as awareness of them enters my meditative awareness. I will draw minimal conclusions, but there is vast learning that always comes with meditation and I share according to my personal nature. There are many aspects which cannot be put into words.

After a few sessions (at 0009) I started recording the mantra used, as different mantras have a different energy. When I started this project it was not intended to be a book, but as it grew, it seemed to be a valuable thing to share and I put other writing on hold to share this. You will see a big increase in methodology as I proceed to do sessions. The beginning few sessions have the nature of poetic commentary and then the methodology is refined to present a clear exposition to be shared.

As you read, I hope you will find time to set aside in daily life to meditate and see for yourself the benefits. I am an advocate for engaging a life in the society of humanity and not withdrawing in any way. Meditation is a tool for living a fuller and richer life through knowing the sacred mystery of yourself at a deeper and more truthful level.

Session 0001:

I experience that Consciousness is like a field and all sensory data enters it and leaves it. The field of Consciousness is the unifying basis and perceives all the sensory data. In meditation my thoughts become much less frequent and in the time between thoughts I am my Consciousness and sensory data still enters me, the field of my awareness, and passes through and is gone. While I can sense the remaining vibrations as memory and call them into a thought process, the majority pass through and are gone.

Images arise, such as seeing my 2.0 Jinashi Shakuhachi flute and sensing I should focus on playing that instrument, from among my other Shakuhachi flutes. Therefore I receive guidance for my active daily life. This guidance is not the main experience of meditation, but rather one of many ancillary benefits. Meditation facilitates improving one's functional life and actually attaining a more holistic and balanced life, but remember there is a deeper aspect which must be experienced and has amazing numinous benefits.

Session 0002:

I contemplate that true Tantra (living life to the fullest and most rewarding possible extent) is the activity of weaving Mantra through Consciousness to form awareness of the Mystery of the tapestry of life.

I have the visualization that Mantra is like a violin bow and the instrument is my body. The Breath moves the Mantric bow across the strings of my being and the place where the bow and strings touch and engage in the dance of unity is my Heart and from there the radiant sound of the glow of the field of Consciousness shines with clarity, illuminating the Mystery. The glorious Consciousness unites with the sacred Mystery of form (physical, mental, emotional, astral, etc.) in a supreme Union.

Mantra is like the breath blowing upon the edge of the Shakuhachi flute. The Mantra touches the ever current edge of time and specific currents flow into the flute of form and resonates with specific energies, to resonate and weave a song. The player and the notes remain on the current edge of time, the boundary where form continually transforms, but merge into the song's energy and follow the flow.

The heart is like the sun and the breath is like the moon and these four are each a cycle, a vibration with a unique timeline or a dimension of time binding us. Multiple cycles of vibration weave together and the field of Consciousness is steady, still, and silent as the threads of time pass through us. **Time is not linear, it is multiple cycles which overlap and form multi-dimensional ripples and these patterns manifest as a spiraling fractal of time.**

Session 0003:

In the vast openness of being as Consciousness, in the inner space of awareness, the body is suspended in the surrounding essence of being. The mind stops for a few breaths and then there arises a vision and then thoughts consider the impression which are felt as the vision leaves awareness and then thoughts quiet for some breaths and a new vision arises so subtly that the thoughts that arise seem almost to be stand alone, but they are based on the vision or subtle form which arises first. Then a melody arises and like the vision it brings forth some feelings, an awareness which follows it through time, holding on to the passing notes, for in the here and now there is only the current tone, while the song requires recollection, the memory aspect of mind.

Returning to the open space, where all thoughts have ceased and the mantra flows naturally with the breath as they merge and both ride the same cycle of momentum which is living spirit. The body is transparent and the space of awareness embraces it as other sounds in the environment also come and go. There is an indescribable feeling which the body imprints upon the field of awareness and it has a color, sound, or taste of the unique flavor of my being. There is awareness of the inner fire, which warms and maintains the rich texture of the transparent bodily form which floats in the higher dimensional field of awareness. The sense of warmth and completeness seems nourishing and the discomfort of my toothache is absent.

Commentary 01:

This brings forth a post meditation question, 'What specifically arises?'. As in dreams there is sometimes a correlation to one's life, either a past event bubbling up into the present dream in some mutated form or a precognitive energy. Sometimes the images and then the attendant mental thoughts have a vividness, as in the story of comparing meditation to playing music above, and other times seem somewhat random and sometimes even absurd (such as an image of a fork and the wondering about if old food remains between the times – how absurd and irrelevant is that(?)).

While we have a spirit which has intent and will-power to choose and some ability to control, the impressions which arise are not personally chosen. One can set an intent and manufacture images to arise, yet unbidden images from the mystery of images flowing into one's awareness is worthy of contemplation. Mentally I can assume that many of them reflect something in my global mental field with its vast catalog of past impressions (perhaps I saw a dubious fork come out of the dishwasher without really thinking about it (?)), yet things arise which I cannot easily ascribe to my own mental assemblage (my mind in its totality). **There seems to be another ordering will or subconscious persona which affects the flow, for in some way it is not pure chaos, but rather it reflects me or teaches me by revealing something I would not think about.**

Session 0004:

Falling into the silence with the mantra and my breath, I get an image of a sphere surrounded by blackness and around that is a white pixelated mist with an irregular boundary and the sphere momentarily gains color so that I know it is the Earth globe and then the misty region closes in and obscures the sphere. I return to the silence and clear astral screen and meditate for a while more, when this image repeats and therefore has some intrinsic meaning for me to grasp.

It is normal for many astral images to arise as images similar to hypnagogic or hypnopompic images, but in a manner in which the observing Consciousness is clear that they are non-physical and that the mind can consider an associated meaning. If thoughts arise during meditation, one returns to mantra, but significant thoughts are accepted for a few breaths. **If the same image appears more than once, it should be contemplated as there is some precedence in the importance of a message in the image.**

In the space where my thoughts have stopped and there is just being and breathing mantra becomes automatic, my body seems like a boundary of a container and the inner space is vibrating very rapidly, much faster than the breath or heart beat rhythms. This appears to be causing the boundary to vibrate as well, though slightly slower and more as if rippling. The vibration moves to the space outside the boundary, but seems to dissipate rapidly in the more open and less energy dense space.

What should I make of mist descending upon the Earth and obscuring it? We have the tale that when the Younger Dryas catastrophe and flood happened, that a mist went up from all the land and the sky could not be perceived as separate from the Earth. The surviving humans scrabbled about in a deep fog looking for food during the forty years of it raining day and night. Perhaps just a mythological tale, but the oceans did rise by a large amount and that was accompanied by a thousand year cold spell, a disaster and global extinction event. Is the meditation vision somehow reflecting the clouds falling to Earth in this past epoch, or is it just a genetic scar or psychic trauma passed down reminding us of the disaster that occurred; or is it a warning?

Meditation brings forth some images that can be very symbolic and therefore contemplated with many layers of meaning. **It is my hopefulness for a glorious human future that I am motivate to do this work of writing this book.** Although time erases everything, life and the human species passes continuous threads into the future in amazing ways. Eventually all things written will be erased by time, but the impressions imprinted in human consciousness will remain as the changes steer human history.

Session 0005:

The sense of my field of Consciousness projects through the auditory field which is surrounding my being and I have the awareness of sounds in various positions in the world around me. I get the sense of my body as another field which is perceived as surrounding and encompassing the central origin of Consciousness. Then as the astral vision comes, I can see my body from different perspectives. The astral vision seems to originate and be located in my third eye, or through my forehead and into a vast space of visual phenomena. Yet I can be aware of the heart center and the lower areas of the body. There remains some presence of intent arising to direct focus, and yet the energies that exist within the field of awareness are existent of themselves and it is one aspect of Consciousness to focus and be concentrated where phenomena exist.

There is the time of releasing where the mantra on the breath becomes so automatic it fades into the breath and there is open space. Whether the mantra is cycling above or below, one pole remains open and in that pause there still exists presence. I vaguely sensed the difference of the right side and left side of the field of awareness and this seems significant. Scientifically we know parity is not conserved: left and right can be determined as specific properties of our material realm which can be determined as distinct. Above and below as well as in front and behind also have unique qualities to be explored. These three variations in the field resolve in the chest, referred to as the heart. This sub-center of gravity is where I experience the flow of subtle energy into and out of my Consciousness.

Toward the end of my meditation as I was slowly coming back to waking awareness, I felt my feet touching each other. I knew they were flat on the floor, yet the sensation of exchanging warmth through touch existed. I observed the sensations and then finally moved my feet slightly, confirming they were flat on the floor and not touching. Interesting that I experienced a tactile sensation which was not physical, but which felt physical to my conscious awareness. **The astral of**

dreaming body seems completely real in all sensory data when one is consciously present in it with lucid awareness.

Session 0006:

Ra-Ma, Ram-Ma, Ha-Ri Si-Ta, Ha-Ri Si-Ta, Si-Ta Si-Ta, Ha-Ri Ha-Ri, ...

(occasional: Hari Radha, Hari Radha, Radha, Radha, Hari, Hari)

Siti Ram, See-Tah, Rham, ...

First vision was of a clear glass spray mist bottle, with a gentle push spray from the top, blowing into my face, refreshing, but shocking. Then a sense of me meditating and being brought into full awareness of my naked body as a bucket of water was pouring over my head, and then being offered a blanket for warmth, and also as a covering to reassert my privacy. Then meditating in the desert in the morning heat, and when really hot having a bucket of cold water poured over my head again, shocking and yet invigorating/exciting. Then the contemplation that a bucket of water is extreme, and a mist spray in the face of cool water would suffice. Then the touching of my forehead as the meditator followed by a misting. Of course I was sitting in my living room in a comfortable chair the whole time.

All these rituals seeming very sensual, yet spiritual in the sense of integrating awareness at multiple levels. I report these visuals as in some ways happening to me on a deeper sensual level and yet in some ways happening simultaneously to a woman somewhere else. There is a sense of the goddess (or universal creative energy) amid the presence of the Godhead (supreme sentient consciousness. as well as personal Consciousness). There is also a sense of a Goddess as a person. This mantra uses the names of Goddesses, so therefore brought forth these sensations.

I am starting to take more notes as I continue this personal experiment of documentation. Amid the visuals, which I do not report and sometimes do not remember in my usual mode of meditation, there is a very sensual nature to meditation. One's body is embedded in Consciousness and is subtly illuminated, vibrantly alive, pleasantly inflamed, and mysterious such that it asks the question, 'What is the true nature of being alive and being blessed to have a body?'. **The meditation experience invites and insights one to look at life and brings a desire to live more fully.**

Visions must have continuity and either repeat or chain together and tell a story or follow a logical contemplative narrative to be worth remembering and reporting. One must note that while the dialog seems to flow, each vision or vision sequence is separated by many breaths of mantra. The entire meditation in this case was thirty or forty minutes (for someone's first few years it is recommended one does a twenty minute session); while in the meditative state I do not sense the passage of time and since I did not look at a clock I can only guess at the duration. Vision or word stories (thoughts) arise and fade and one must imprint them in memory in order for them to have future reference. It is similar to knowing one was dreaming a lot in a night, but not having details except when some poignant or absurd element makes the dream stick and it is remembered in the morning.

Also, like dreams, if a vision or a thought arises which was triggered by events or conditions in one's daily life, it might be ignored and not worth reporting. Such triggered thoughts would only have value to this study if a following vision or chain of thoughts provided a new and unique insight which had not occurred in daily life. Initial visions of a mighty warrior with a feline face and a petite hypersensitive goddess were not reported because they originated in having read the Ramayana.

One focus here is the nature of what arises, what falls into one's conscious awareness. From where it falls will remain a mystery (as perhaps the mythical word descriptions of a sub consciousness or a super-sentient source), though it is a question worth contemplating. I intend to give more focus to intention and what effect intention has on the experience. When meditating the experience is not prone to control, yet in life we have intention and can carry intention into the meditation.

In proofreading I am adding this note that after a few more sessions I will report everything in detail and in sequence, contrary to this initial intent. These session will span two years, since going into a deep astral meditation is a very intense art and each meditation of this type will need to be contemplated and assimilated before the next session. I meditate daily and the mantra used evolves and must be used for a week or three until it is so assimilated that it takes no effort, but has its own momentum and requires no effort.

Session 0007:

Aham (I Am) (In-breath Ahh , out-breath-Hum).

A bit with out-breath Hoom and some use of Ihum (In-breath: long Ee, out=breath: Hoom).

It should first be noted that internal sound is much more versatile than speech, in that the number of sounds that the mind is able to bring forth vastly exceeds any spoken language due to the physical limitations of the bodies organs of speech. As the mantra gains momentum, such that one does not have any intent driving it, it becomes as natural as breath, and the sound will often resolve itself into a natural internal quality. This is an additional topic for this experiential research, which is motivated by my desire to understand. Hoom and Hum are similar and neither vocal word captures it.

The first visual was of Zen shakuhachi flute music script, a single vertical line progressing. I mention this because at that point I may have been able to pick up a pen and write it as it scrolled down, but decided to continue meditating. Reading in a descending vertical line seems like a natural process once one learns to read shakuhachi music and reading music is similar to the passage of time. Therefore this is worth noting that astral images scroll by with time and tell a story. **Reading is similar to video or watching living motion in that a story flows by.** I did not recognize the musical piece and so there was creative energy (referred to as Shakti) generating it.

The next visual was of a woman's face, very beautiful, but somewhat artistically presented as an astral Image. As I felt attraction and then the face morphed to a man's face, thus eliminating any sexual energy (since I am a heterosexual male). This sequence repeated itself several times. I might interpret this to imply that the faces were not to generate human emotion, but more to express the duality within the unity of internal space. The logical inference would be that 'I' as the observer conscious of the images was not seeing them as aspects of my own creative energy, but rather as having some external reality. Consciousness is not of any form, but all form perceived passes through it. Indeed, I followed this phase with the intent to connect with spiritual beings and the faces morphed, but if there was a transmission from spiritual beings in this phase of the meditation, I cannot discern it or describe it with words, I was just watching.

In addition to these images and several other images, was the sense of my body as a space. I mean that I was inside of my body and it was not hollow, but neither was its definition the boundaries that are ordinarily conceived. I can sense my entire form and at times moved my attention to 'light up' specific body areas (volumes) as if it were a 3-D object suspended in my Consciousness. Aham (I Am) is considered a 'Sacred Heart' mantra and in this sense the internal space of my being was emphasized. I had little awareness of sounds around me.

Early in the meditation I switched briefly to Ihum and that connected my inner space to my outer space, pulsing with my breath. With Aham I was internal, in my body cave. This leads me to conclude that for self-healing Aham is a very proficient mantra. My body Consciousness was not on a physical level and my awareness of toothache pain faded from my awareness. After the meditation, it was much less pronounced. Ihum by contrast radiated energy outward and should be used when someone has internal flow and can connect to another person to do healing work.

Final thoughts on my form suspended in my Consciousness, which sounds like a duality, but in actuality there was only the experiential perception. I was both inside and all around my body and the body was part of me. It was not experienced as other, though the thinking mind and our language works on that basis. As I breathe, the focus of attention flows with In-Breath descending and out-breath ascending. This micro-cosmic orbit does not imply that awareness did not completely coincide with all experience and the total bodily form. This is hard for the mind to grasp and this points to the experiential reality being much richer and more complex that words can describe.

The feeling of being in meditation is not really accurately described by visual imagery or any story in words. As one breaths air, the air itself is invisible, and so deeply innate to daily existence that it is rarely in our awareness as it always exists. All the internal qualities of my body, its unique and peculiar nature cannot be accurately described as color, sound, taste, smell, or other external sensory categories. It can be poetically said to be a whole symphony. **Just like the smell of spring air, words only point to the experience for those who have experienced it and otherwise does not contain the nuance intended.** The inability of the mind to analyze and quantify all the components of being in an experience is due to words being symbols of low dimensionality.

Implicit in Aham is my unique ray of Consciousness, my vibrational frequency beyond any notion of higher or lower frequency, but rather as a tone with many complex overtones defining a timbre, tone color, or tone quality which is me. Being is radiantly vibrant and when resting in Aham there is personal healing through resting in the essence of I Am.

The greater 'I AM', the divine Consciousness ('i am' that 'I AM') is an inherent quality of the sacred mystery captured in this Sanskrit phrase of the ongoing divine creative energy from which personal 'i am' is derived. In a later age this was added to the old testament as the reference to the supreme divine which is sustaining me and every living thing in space-time. The aham 'i am' of personal consciousness is potentiated by the Aham 'I AM' of universal consciousness. The ever-changing dynamic present cosmic dance of changes deposits impressions in consciousness. In meditation time has a different flow and as I settle into the aham Aham, there exists something (but not a thing) which is beyond time, which is my essence and which is divine essence. It is settling into this liminal essence as a unified whole, which is present in time and yet is somehow beyond time, which balances or re-tunes my being and this meditation process is the heart of healing.

Session 0008:

Paravati (2 breaths: Out-breath Pa/Par, In-Breath Ra/Ah; out-breath Va/vah, in=breath Ti (as Tea).

Para means supreme and Vati has many meanings (air, garden, damp, moon,...). Even though Parvati is the Goddess name, but in this meditation I worked with Paravati, 'supreme vital energy'. This grammatical contemplation of my variation is after the meditation and rightly so, since I was simply attracted to the thought sounds described and followed my intuition. Paravati could also be conceived of as a reference to 'Blowing Zen' or playing the sacred music on a Shakuhachi flute.

Initially the syllables were with quick breaths (slightly faster than normal, not deep meditation breathing), and did not pull me into the astral, but kept me grounded. The breathing was focused on my center of gravity, (Chinese Dan Tien, Japanese Hara), which the female body surrounds with the Womb, but is the lower axis of breath for all humans and animals. This brought me to the realization that the mantra was referring to the Womb of all creation. This is the place where souls of Consciousness enter into form to be born. It is also said that an opening or crack forms around the center of gravity and this is the gate of death through which the soul departs. Therefore the state of my Consciousness was embodied physically. A brief visual of a stylized eye with eye lashes looking down from over my head signified to me that this was a meditation on the supreme Womb, the form which holds all Consciousness, the Consciousness of all beings, and therefore my Consciousness.

I gradually felt all the 'a/ah' sounds softening (none sounding like the 'a' in father). This took a fair amount of time (perhaps 10-15 minutes) to shift in my meditation. During the first phase my bodily pain from a toothache increased, but then as the 'a's softened and my breath finally got deeper I was pain free. I was now connected to my higher energetic form, but still remained very physical. I heard the dog snoring and the birds outside chirping, desiring me to fill the feeder with seed as I do in the mornings. I heard the traffic in the distance and then a road grader went slowly by, grinding the dirt road in front of our house. I thought of the demands made upon women to care for others, the children and the elderly, and to cook and clean and on and on. Then my stomach gurgled several times, wanting breakfast, and I realized that Paravati, the Cosmic Womb, the form and energy of the entire Cosmos, calls to Consciousness with a need, a longing, a quintessential desire. I had first started with a few breaths of Uma, but quickly switched to Paravati as the mantra for this session, so I was already meditating when this mantra called to me.

Finally I got to an astral phase and my bodily form was suspended in spatial Consciousness and appeared red. Then the only other images received were as a blue female face, non-distinct, and then a female body in blue light. These were very sublime images and my emotions flitted through responses, such as worship, devotion, sexual energy, nurturer energy, motherly energy, but none fit the energy of the vibration of Paravati. Finally I arrived at service. **The Cosmos is breeding/evolving ever more conscious life forms. Therefore the work of one in harmony with the Womb of the Cosmos and her energy is to be acting in service to raising the Consciousness.** The blue merged into my red as if both existed together, viewed as vibrating pixelated intermingling, not dissolving into each other. I realize I am both creative spirit manipulating the cosmic energy and form through choices of activity, as well as the Consciousness which illuminates it to receive awareness of the Mystery in greater and greater degrees. **This then appears as the lesson, both for me personally and as guidance for what humanity should consider its main focus: becoming more conscious to be better co-creators.**

Commentary 02:

There was no premeditated plan up to this point, but I am settling into a defined methodology to continue. For fifty years I have meditated with spontaneity, sometimes sticking to one mantra, either only one breath (Bija or seed mantra) or short chant mantras of several words/breaths. Now I am now focused on exploring mantra from an energetic perspective and so am seeking to dedicate these documented meditations to a single mantra (Bija or Chant) in my thoughts with my breath. I have the assumption that the sound vibration affects my Consciousness' vibration through resonance. Some association from a concept of word meaning creeps into the meditation, but it is my desire to be so present with the vibrational form of the sound of the thought, that I experience and come to understand the vibrational energy itself. The 'thought sound' itself creates with a specific vibratory nature or quality and imparts a feeling and a teaching which is on a much higher dimension than thinking, reasoning, or mental informational constructs.

Session 0009:

The toothache was severe and I was not able to meditate, I sought distraction in activity. Fortunately I had an appointment in the afternoon to get it extracted. This experience was also a spiritual lesson about mortality and human frailty. I am reminded to always be compassionate toward others. Not everyone will have the self-control to meditate. Physical, mental, and emotional circumstances can make settling into the silence with breath and mantra difficult. I am humbled to never imagine I am more than human, but rather to know that to be human is a miraculous gift. I am humbled to know that being able to meditate is a blessing and does not make me more spiritual, only acting with compassionate love is spiritual. Meditation is a phenomenal tool for both taming the unruly mind to allow very deep thinking and also a tool for exploring and healing one's life journey.

Session 0010:

Shakti Shiva Shakti Shiva Shiva Shiva Shakti Shakti (Out-breath: Shahk, In-Breath: Tea, Out-breath: She, In-Breath: Vah ...)

    I began with Shakti, added Shiva and soon thereafter I arrived at this mantra in the maha mantra pattern. Being eight breaths, it has powerful momentum. One of the first images to become visible was of an upside down forest, which caused some precipitation of thoughts. **Shakti is the Spirit, the creative energy which condenses into the whole Cosmos moving as a play, while Shiva is Consciousness.** The play of all things is a reflection of the original Spirit, the Word as the primary vibration which underlies all of the ever- changing dance of life. Reflections are reversed in our Consciousness as it penetrates into the mystery and revealing it, is seeing inside-out. Meditating deeper I got the sense that my conscious Shiva light which touches and engages with the play of life, is witnessing the Shakti mystery of the Cosmos and is really an aspect of the Shakti, the Spirit weaving the play.

    This meditation was somewhat transcendental, as I was not aware of my body suspended in my Consciousness, nor of the outside world. The momentum of the mantra brought me into a blissful state and yet a very aware state, where there was freedom and the present edge of time was predominant. I was more aware of the mantra, than the breath. If one is outside looking in, then the paradigm of a conscious observer and the thought-sound of the mantra as observed merge into aspects of being, of just actively observing, similar to how the senses all merge into a single sense of our being journeying in the world. The union of Shiva, the light of Consciousness, and the active creative Spirit of the Word manifesting as the vibrations, the changes, the dance of Shakti, is so natural and seamless that it is only in the inside-out reflection which the mind creates that duality exists. In the meditation, when this dichotomy, which the mind creates dissolves, one is just blissful experiencing and both the perceiver (experiencer) and perceived (experience) are in unity (just perceiving, just experiencing), for one cannot exist without the other because they are only dual in mental analysis.

Session 0011:

HamSa (Out-breath Hum, In-Breath Sah).

Saturday morning and my wife was busy around the house and I probably picked up some of the busyness, as my mind kept returning to things to do and thoughts to follow up on. There were very few visuals. This mantra has been referred to as Shiva's breath (creation and destruction, condensing and releasing) and did seem very connected to breath and perhaps mimics Aham (I Am) and both as related to Sa-Ah which is said to be the sound of breath. The mantra SoHam is a related form.

In Hamsa the Out-Breath (Hum) containing additional quality of release, as giving and nurturing energy. I found a very different energy if I associated the syllables, breaths, as HamSa rather than SaHam (not changing out-breath Hum and In-Breath Sah, but my mental association of the word with breath. Which part of the word was the second syllable caused focus on that part of breath and therefore the focus was in the upper pause (HamSa) or the lower pause (SaHam). **It is in the pauses between the In-Breath and Out-Breath that there is opportunity to know energetic-awareness more fully.** Note that this is very profound and deep wisdom. The phase of transition is a thin place, a space where time shifts.

Movement between the lower center of gravity (of the whole body) and the upper center of gravity (of or above the head) circles around the heart center (of the chest), but this mantra kept focus on breathing and its cycling in this session. Each meditation has a resonance in the mantra used against one's vibrating energetic body and so each meditation session may provide more insight if one is deeply engaged.

Session 0012:

SAUH: Out-breath sound descending (Sah), In-breath ascending with (uhhh).

Sacred Heart mantra breathing horizontally rather than the vertical micro-cosmic orbit. This is blissful more than ecstatic. The flow of energy coming from the deepest essence in the chest area of the energy body (Visarga) and streaming forth in loving energizing service to bless others. While my form floats within Consciousness, the waves are from within and flowing out to nurture. Several times I sensed parts of my body also receiving healing vibrations, adjustments of energies which are not pleasant, nor painful, but have an intensity.

There was a great deal of cosmic presence in the meditation. **There are many beings on the higher vibrational dimension of the telepathic web.** By vibrating above the mundane human level, my thoughts stilled and became very thin. At times my breath also became very slow and soft and the mantra kept it going as I reached deeper levels while maintaining awareness. The first cosmic presence was the Queen Devi who seems to have available attention and strong interest, though I suspect she can maintain multiple awareness threads. Her awareness is revealing and penetrates my space completely and yet I invited her to ride along, since I was only sending forth the deep waters of life through my Sacred Heart (Hriyadam). I only requested of her to bless the other meditators on Earth who are also connected into the telepathic web. This journey was not visual, but I entered into the visual with her eyes and then briefly let astral images dance as kaleidoscopic white light in the reddish black field.

I then desired the perfume of the sweetest essence of the Blue Devi, the wild one who contains superb vitality and immense power. Although she has luscious form, I recalled a dream from the night before and her eyes which became a powerful attraction. I did not smell her most desirous heavenly fragrance, better than any floral or perfumed scent of the Earthly realm, but there was the most subtle teasing hint of it. Telepathically she indicated I would catch the scent at the most appropriate times in my life and she would therefore teach me through this essence. The whole time I was still horizontally transmitting energy from my heart.

The third astral meditating sentient being to make its presence known was bird like. The first two were very high masters, but this being was more grounded in a life. I imagine the first two may have some sort of physical existence, but exist primarily in the subtler dimensions where even the astral realms are a lower level. The bird like being was curious and seemed to have a duty in the higher dimensions, a sort of guardian. I accepted its presence with a neutral attitude, but put forth that it should not change the energy and should be of service to the meditators of Earth. I assume that everyone needs blessings and send my energy to everyone, but communion with higher beings requires total mental and emotional visibility and many of those incarnate on Earth would cringe at being totally revealed in the light, naked down to their soul.

While my intent was to be of service to the other humans who meditate, I also was accepting of their energy and their commitment to meditating. The relational energy allowed me to be aware at a very deep and profound level. There is indeed a multiplier effect when a group meditates together and the more people meditating upon the Earth, the more that everyone's energy is refined. The blue throat of Shiva (Consciousness both individual and supreme) is the consumption of the poison of our ancestral trauma and our personal trauma by the supreme light. We are refined in the very act of sitting in meditation, being our consciousness, and holding the intent of commitment to spiritual awakening to greater awareness. **We are never alone or disconnected, there is nothing private or hidden from the celestial beings.**

Commentary 03:

Note that post meditation perspective is a valid overlay to being there. What or who is encountered is not to imply there is a physical existence to these Angelic Beings, nor to deny it. Rather to report that there is an astral (dreaming) reality which is both a reflection of my current state of being in life and also, I hypothesize some deeper sentience. One can think it is my own being or accept that higher conscious beings are influencing the perceived astral journey: I cannot determine this from my visioning and do not spend time contemplating what I do not have the data to determine.

As the perceiver I must be very clear that in all cases, all of our daily engagement with the world, which is a subjective filter over a vast and inconceivable quantum reality, is better termed the Mystery. As a mortal human there are many things I cannot understand and humans have had Goddess, Gods, Angels, or other spiritual beings as part of their lives for all of known history. The vast majority of humans on Earth live in this paradigm, even since the religion of materialism has become the academic standard. The Mystery is the quantum realm embedded in the Planck Sea of primal Vibration and gas many layers of ordering, of informational structural relationships, which subsume each other and constitute the totality, the Cosmos, within which ever more powerful sentient beings evolve.

The human sense of a material world is created from very limited sensory bands perceived by our bodies and all plants and animals live in different realities. I deeply honor science as a methodology, but not as a belief system or religion of materiality, and therefore I am doing this more formal reporting of experiences which meditation offers. From this point forward I will seek to be more detailed and list more of the perceptions which can be described in the symbols of words. Language does not exist for much of this.

Session 0013:

SAUH: Out-breath sound descending (Sah), In-breath ascending with (uhhh).

I started with presenting an initial invitation to beings more conscious than I, who were aware within the telepathic web, the subtle reality, to provide teachings that were aligned with the sentience of the Cosmos. I recognize that the ultimate cosmic sentience is directly accessible, yet teachers are always good. One of the first images I received was of a Caucasian woman wearing glasses and who was a scholar. I had an impression that the imagery was of my wife, but while meditating the presence seemed more mystical and had a different inner quality and indeed each of us has a more mystical reality and inner quality than we naturally assume in our daily roles.

One reoccurring image, which I also saw yesterday. was of pages of text. This lets me know that while I am reading books, the actual image being imprinted within my being is text arranged on a page. Text is, at this point in time, humanities most powerful symbolic reflection of the Mystery, though western text is very limited in its linear and logical nature, except when used poetically. In meditation there was only the visual perception, not this analysis, but the text changed from standard English to a character based language like Asian characters which is ordered vertically and from right to left (similar to the shakuhachi flute music which I read).

This image was of calligraphic characters in black upon an enameled surface, at first like a spoon holder, but then as a sheet designed for holding text. It changed to Honkyoku Japanese Shakuhachi flute music and then back to characters in an unknown language. I again saw the woman and she was a scholar in this language and so not my wife, but symbolically represented the request for a teacher I had presented. At this age in life I do not seek to take up learning such a language, as fascinating as it is. This is a powerful lesson in how intent can direct a meditation and override the innate vibrational resonance spontaneous arising with the input which the specific thought sound has.

I also was periodically aware of the Queen Devi for whom I had intent to be present as a teacher or invited as an observer. I then had an apologetic intent, as I did not want to consume her valuable time, feeling unworthy as a primitive human, but she conveyed that she was part of a group network of minds and had many streams of perception available. In that case any individual body was a component in providing its set of multiple perceptual streams and could not be considered as an individual in the manner that we humans consider ourselves and yet was an individual experiencer. She stayed in the background as presence. Of course one can analyze this as being my own 'higher self' if one wishes, but that is just the mind shifting terms. I am referring to a divine presence which is available in meditation. I do not think personification is reality, but it is the nature of our understanding as human personalities and also of language which seeks to associate a specific feeling of a sentient presence with a characterization or personality.

There was a phase where I saw my body naked in a recliner, as if I was looking out of my eyes, rather than from above or the side. This was curious as I was not ever naked in my recliner in the living room. Then I saw a woman's body from this perspective and yet after a moment of focus realized this was not my body transformed, but my Consciousness being presented a different perceptual stream. Perception of a woman's body inherently generates sexual energy in a heterosexual male and this gave the perception that I was inside my body floating in the sea of my Consciousness. I was not perceiving my being as inside my physical body, but rather both inside and outside of it as a larger field of awareness. There is a very powerful spiritual energy transcendent to my awareness of being within my sensual field of perception and my bodily presence. The mantra remained heart centered and the other aspects or channels of perception were always less than or floating on top of another layer of sensory input.

Commentary 04:

   As the meditation concluded I found myself more in my thoughts and slowly slipping out of the astral realm. In a sense I could say that meditation has qualities which are similar to a 'Waking Induced Lucid Dream' (WILD) in that one is conscious and awake, yet is dipping into the astral-dream levels of mental capability. It would seem that many artists, engineers, physicists, and other creative people have some connection to the art of being visionaries, yet the act of meditation is beyond the momentary flash of inspiration and is an ongoing conscious practice which enhances one's ability in whatever one engages in during one's daily life in the world. Renunciation and asceticism have no value. Meditation is a way to charge one's daily life with both a peacefulness and a vitality which work together for making a more full life. Generally my meditations last 20 or 30 minutes. This journaling is much more time consuming than the practice itself, but is an expression of my nature as a writer.

   Later in the evening while listening to a podcast with my eyes closed and being aware of my breathing, I had an astral vision of a wall of books. I thought that I have a lot of books when I had bought more today. Then I was in a small room with the walls covered in bookshelves full of books. A woman, that was a cartoon-like librarian, indicated I should look up and the walls covered in books went up many stories. Perhaps I have read that many books. I have been considering that although I enjoy reading and gain from it, I wonder if mental contemplation leads anywhere (?). Here I am writing and perhaps this will be a book or available text, but what I have received cannot be offered in words beyond inspiring others to Trip on Meditation. Books have changed the course of my life and I hope that I inspire meditation because it offers people more talent in life and a freedom which brings inner peace.

Session 0014:

Aim: as in Aym: out-breath Aye, In-Breath mmm

    This is supposed to be the mantra of Adya Shakti and Sarasvati, but I did not have the Adya Shakti connection while doing this. Today was a busy morning and I did not feel this meditation deeply as the energy of the Cosmos. The meditation brought me into a peaceful state. As Sarasvati is the Goddess of wisdom and learning, as well as music and arts, I will note that I kept returning to various letter symbols and conceiving of how they look on the page. I got into imaging the Japanese Shakuhachi flute music scripts, of which there are several variations that share commonality, while others are different enough that they must be learned as a new script. I am starting to learn Hitorogiri flute which shares symbols, but not the fingerings or notes. For a long time a symbolic language for Just Intonation has been percolating within me and I am motivated to create it. The thoughts and images of this musical notation system kept arising and that is fine. Different meditations are expected to go in different directions.

    It should be noted that the Word (Vak) represented often as AUM (another double vowel mantra, as is Aim) is said to be at the core of the Shakti, the primal energy, which creates, orders, propels, and transforms the entire Cosmos. Symbolic representation through Bija (seed) mantra is one's way of sharing in and co-creating with the primal energy. The seed contains the blueprint for the entire plant, as the letters for words, and then forming thoughts and all the intricacies of mental comprehension and philosophy and belief. Therefore a new musical notation may lend itself to a new exploration of Raga, which is more than scales and modes, but also contains detailed motifs which express the character and Rasa, the emotional feel or flavor of the music. The energy of the mantra did apparently express itself as Sarasvati, goddess of writing and music, and was about manifesting rather than experiencing deeper dimensional realms.

Session 0015:

Sarasvati: out-breath: Sah, In-Breath Rah, out-breath Svah, In-Breath Tee.

A very nice and healing meditation which really slowed me down. Even though it is morning, my thoughts want to contemplate so many potential doings for the day, but they quickly subsided to the occasional arising and the arising was not about today's lists, but did sometimes included future activity. There were several times when my breathing became very shallow, almost like I was not breathing and this meant the syllables of thought sound were not easily in awareness and so I would consciously breath deeper and take some very slow breaths. I have encountered this in other meditations, but it was very shallow several times. I wondered if I was getting enough air, but I was comfortable and my Consciousness was lucid.

The only visual was of a woman's face, but always different, both in bone structure and in expression. The face was generally in a blue light upon the dark background and so had an amorphous quality. The expression was sometimes serious. sometimes blissful, sometimes curious, and other such expressions. The structure or genetic form of the face seemed to change as if to express the emotion better. It was always calm and reassuring, as if expressing a teaching due to caring about me.

I asked for a teaching and then saw this 'asking' was me being needy and wanting. I asked to be of service, but what service would be most helpful I do not know, and I did not want to be a burden. I asked for help with our crashing civilization, but again, that is me requesting energy. Overall, I started to release my need for energy exchange and neither sought to give nor receive, but just to be there in the unfolding of time in a natural manner, without my mind's wanting to receive or my mind's wanting to provide. This is a good relational state which is healthy and balanced: just being is what meditation should be. The need to get or receive implies putting expectation on the future. Being present in exchange without expectation is the balanced way to live. Post meditation I can say this is a very powerful teaching.

During the meditation I also experienced my body in the field of Consciousness, but it had less of a visual quality and more of a tactile quality. It was not physical, heavy and bound by gravity while sitting in a chair, in the same way as other meditations, but its overall form had a sensual quality, as if a subtle vibration were causing a radiance of some indescribable bliss. It was not sexual, but rather the whole body was alive and full of some vibrant energy of peacefulness, as paradoxical as vibrant power combined with peaceful bliss may sound. It was the feeling of being fully alive and yet calm and serene. This also seemed to be an essential quality that the astral face always had amid all its changes.

My final note is about the sound of the syllables or sounds. Sah, Rah, and Svah are all similar and core letter sounds. Ti (tee as in tea) has an ascending quality. I tried briefly to reverse which syllables went with which part of the breath, but was quickly reverted to the above orientation. Several times I was attracted to the richness of the first three sounds which seemed very grounding and nourishing; and then the Ti had an addition of refinement and was ascending. None of the syllables seemed to want to be the accented or become a dominant one, but they danced in balance.

Session 0016:

Om Parvati: Out-Breath Om (Ohhmmm/aaauuummm) and In-Breath Parvati (Par-vah-Tee).

Using the whole Goddess name as a Triple In-Breath is something I learned after about ten years of practicing mantra. **There is a natural triplet nature to an in-breath.** I first worked with sacred Christian mantras and had an ascension philosophy which took me a long time to deprogram from my conditioning. In this case having the OM/AUM as an Out-Breath seemed balanced. Even though I note this as OM, in my thoughts it had the 'au' quality of AUM. **One will find that upon entering into true meditation, the thought sound vibration is much richer than a language, spoken words, or the symbols of letters can incorporate.**

A word of warning about the imbalance of ascension philosophy is in order. The true purpose of meditation is to become more fully human and to be able to engage life more fully, with greater mental clarity. A desire to escape life, whether based on false notions of escaping suffering, attaining heaven, or escaping reincarnation does not result in a spiritual life, but is a selfish philosophy and also promotes the bigger ego trap of thinking one is better than other people, one is on the one true path, or one is saved. Mediation is a humbling tool which will allow one to work through stuck trauma and come to be more fully one's self. Meditation can be a humbling art since it takes many years to learn to control the wild mind and gain mental clarity. As with any true art, one never achieves some final completion and always learns and improves. **A person who is an artist at meditation is a very functional human who possesses a remarkable degree on inner peace amid the ups and downs of a fully engaged life.**

I became very aware of the pause after the In-Breath and before the Out-Breath and even more of the pause after the Out-Breath and before the In-Breath. These two transition points are very powerful to be aware of. They allow one to be in one's Consciousness. I concentrated on the richness of the thought sound and soon external sound was not catching almost any of my attention. Several times my breath slowed and would almost seem to stop, at which point I would increase my focus on the thought sound in order to make my breath deep again and this again opened the upper and lower transition points.

I only consciously extended the pause points of transition between phases of breath very briefly. The natural pause which occurs by the nature of breath cycle I found was longer when I maintained a high focus on the thought sound of the mantra. The pauses would seem to open up in astral space. This was not a very visual meditation. I briefly saw an owl morph into a woman's face and occasionally just a woman's face, but not with much emphasis. However, during the pause, especially the lower pause, I sensed astral space as if I had gone outside of my usual spatial form and there was open space around me.

Hrim Parvati: Out-Breath Hreem, In-Breath Parvati.

I sensed I needed to modify the thought sound and so switched to an Out-Breath with Hrim. This is an extremely powerful and energizing seed mantra of divine feminine power, of birthing, nurturing, and dying. Although the text I had studied stated this was a spiritual heart (Hridaya) mantra, this clearly was centered for me at the energy center just below the navel (Chinese Dan Tien, Japanese Hara, Hindu third Chakra); This is the center of gravity of the body and the space-time gateway which is surrounded by a woman's womb in females. It is the key power place of breathing for everyone.

A few times the face would briefly appear as powerful and frightening, as if the face of death. The feminine warrioress nature to defend the children and the bloody nature of birth and death arose numerous times. Also a sense or feeling my mortality. While one might consider that an evil power was involved, if that idea rose there was a response in the meditation of assurance and a nurturing energy. Death is not evil, it is a natural blessing, as is our response to defend against it.

It provides a tension and thereby an active and stimulating energy of striving to live fully.

I briefly switched back to Om and the intent to do so was generated by the Parvati thought-sound. One can see how this sound is personified as a Goddess because it has an active energy and influence which one will be in relationship with when meditating with it. One might metaphorically say that it is a specific personality which the totality of Cosmos expresses with sentience. I experienced a reaction to the fierce energy and was reassured that this was one of many forms of the spiritual nature.

I wanted to return to the open space when the lower breath pause after an Out-Breath opened. In this pause one might think that at death, with the final Out-Breath of one's journey, that the upper door is the gate, but it is the center of gravity of the assemblage of the human form which is the tunnel of death. Life enters the Cosmos within the center of gravity within a womb connected to a mother by an umbilical cord and that center of gravity is the same location that the living spirit exits through. The umbilical cord is replaced by the greatest meta-entangled cord of fibers of luminous consciousness when we are born, a gravitational entwinement, and that cord connects us to the Earth until we die. When the space opened after a long full out-breath I did not feel threatened or like death would arrive, but did feel like there was a whole extremely vast realm there, waiting to be explored.

There was briefly the presence of a guardian spirit, a watcher with a head much bigger than mine, scrutinizing me. It did not seem menacing, but there was the total revealing of my being in its presence. Consider being suddenly naked on a stage where one was speaking all the thoughts that one has ever held, as if what is thought of in the illusion of being alone in one's mind is being printed out in a live chat, and yet amazingly I did not sense invasive energy. The mind is naked when one achieves true meditation. Indeed, in my peace I invited the presence to view me and journey along for the meditation, then it was gone. I could not enter the open space with a living body and I suspect it is deeper and more vast that the astral realm of lucid dreaming.

There was the sense that the open space was the vast and extremely fluid realm of the dead. Since Parvati is the power to channel life into the Cosmos and birth it into manifestation and also to nourish it and cultivate it, as well as to attend to the dying process, it makes sense that the connection to the realm of the dead, the key to the gate of the realm of the dead, would be present in the thought-sound of Parvati. I do have some book knowledge of the Goddess Parvati's stories and am only expressing my impressions from this current meditation journey, because in meditation my thinking mind is at rest: this is just reporting experience and not mental beliefs. It is my belief that the names of the Goddesses and Gods are vibrational keys left by very advanced sages for us; to make available the sound vibrational resonance which can teach us and the stories allowed their preservation through many dark ages of humanity, as well as providing some insight into the sacred name's energy. Meditation is indeed a verb and not a noun, it is an active process.

Session 0017:

Lakshmi: Out-Breath: Lahk, In-Breath Shmee

The first sensation was of my whole body pulsating. It was like a head to toe pulse from within to without. The sensation was different than floating in the spatial field of Consciousness and was more of being the field itself and being the body at the same time: non-duality. I did not sense a precedence to anybody center. The out-breath was a surrender with a definite end in the hard K sound. The In-Breath was smooth and nourishing. I did not become aware of the pauses at the transitions, even though they were clearly delineated: the entire four phases of breath were seamless and flowed with natural ease.

When I lost focus, I automatically started again with Shakti and then realizing this in a few breaths, I returned to Lakshmi. These two would go great together as a two breath mantra, but I wanted to keep my focus. I briefly tried adding Shrim, as it is related, but it was too hot and energetic at this time for me. This morning was cold and damp, hovering around freezing, so I had started a fire in our small wood burning stove, to dry the house out. When I used Shrim as an Out-Breath, my already warm body seemed to quickly jump up a few degrees and become uncomfortable. The similarity of Lakshmi and Shakti seems to be paralleled in the vibrational resonance they create, but Lakshmi is gentler.

I only had a few visual impressions, one of drinking a cool glass of water which is a natural response to the heat. It did not seem like an offering to me, but rather as advice to honor drinking lots of water, especially after this meditation. The other image was of a word, perhaps of four characters, but the script kept changing to languages that I could not read. Overall this was a very peaceful and serene blissful energy, without much mental activity. A few thoughts arose, but had little power. I was inspired to send out a few blessings, but generally was just present in the breathing.

The astral plane did open up a few times, very briefly. One time in particular it seemed to hold plant life, as in a lush meadow with some trees. It was almost an invitation and yet I had no sense of ability to move into it. It did not occur to me to seek it or to do anything: I was just in a state of being, of receiving. It seemed the energy of Lakshmi or Shakti did not need to honor or appease any gatekeeper to the open realm. In a sense this open realm presents an enticement, as if being given a glimpse of something delicious, yet not actually being given it. There is no sense of being teased or feelings of trickery, since my state was one of surrender to my being, my breath, and the mantra. I perceived a promise that the other realm (call it paradise, heaven, or transcendence) is the most valuable treasure, the satisfaction of the innate longing which rests behind all longings.

Session 0018:

Ambika: In-Breath Am, Out-Breath Bee, In-Breath Kah, Silent in-breath.

I did not find any associate of breath with Ambika that worked as well as this two breath association did. It flowed very naturally with smooth and gentle stability at this time. Several times during the meditation the mantra 'Om Mani Padme Hum' arose. Perhaps the association was the pause after Hum. Both mantras seem to have momentum which is natural and therefore they easily become effortless.

Yesterday we sold the four pregnant ewes from our small flock of Soay sheep. The Ram will be leaving in a couple of days. We will have three wethers for a while. I kept getting impressions from the ewes as if telepathic questioning, like 'Where are you?', 'Where are we?', 'Why did this happen?'. They are on a nice farm with lots of pasture and as my body ages, I need to simplify life, to let things go. I also sensed a questioning from the wethers who were now without the older ewes: just confusion. The Soay Ram seems self-centered and not connected to the changes. The reason I say this all seemed telepathic, rather than a product of my own subconscious, was that it seemed external and not arising from me during the meditation.

This session indicates how life choices and situations influence one's meditation. This is similar to dreams where the events in life sometimes bubble up into one's dreaming. Although one approaches meditation free of intent, there will arise a combination of one's life's momentum and the resonate quality of the mantra. Ambika, as a mothering energy, implies acceptance of the responsibility for those under one's care, but also the releasing at the appropriate time. A mother must release her children when they are grown to live their own lives and assume their own responsibility and then transitions to a grandmother role. Livestock are a responsibility requiring care and nurturing, Soay sheep have wonderful fleece. Pet are a responsibility requiring a lot of training and care, but are very rewarding parts of a rich life. **Things are not true riches, relationships are.** Death claims all possessions, but energy spent in relationships continues.

Session 0019:

SAUH: In-breath Sow with the dual vowel AU rounding over the upper pause and the visarga 'h', 'Ha' or 'Uh' on the out-breath.

   This is a heart mantra and was definitely centered in the heart. It opened space several times significantly and that is something I am working with. The open astral space does not correspond to the luminous field of Consciousness, which my form is suspended in, but rather seems to also float in the luminous Consciousness. It almost seems as if I could enter astral space like being in a lucid dream, but it was not visual in the ordinary sense, but rather a feeling of space, more similar to an acoustic space. Since this mantra was flowing over the upper pause, the lower pause and lower centers of being was more active. I did not sense sexual energy, but the silver chord seemed to be the portal to astral space. It is as if a vast space is opening within my awareness and around me.
   Several times some sayings arose, more as a narrators voice than as my thought energy. These were like dreams from which you wake, knowing the dreams were present, but the memories are lost upon waking. This reminds me of a hypnotic process, where one is hypnotized and yet retains enough current of awareness to allow dialog with a hypnotist. I therefore intend to have a pen and pad of paper to scratch notes on from this point forward and see how that goes. Memory is a fickle thing and only captures what one finds significant, rather than all the minute details. **Memories change with time, even though the past was written in definitive detail.**

Session 0020:

Aum Mani Padme Hum: Out-Breath Ahh In-Breath Mmm, Out-Breath Ma In-Breath Nee, Out-Breath Pod In-Breath Ma, Out-Breath Hum In-Breath Silence (perhaps 'mm' fading to silence).

I sensed the open space and although I perceived it like dream-space or astral-imaginal space, my body sensed it as if it was an actual dimension. Our Consciousness is embedded within the Cosmos through being embedded within our body and yet our Consciousness subsumes our body and is also exterior to our body. This external consciousness is the sensory view when we are awake, but in meditation it is a field surrounding the perceiver. External sensations, like sound or our dog nosing me to see if she could get attention are inside the Consciousness field. Our dog had intent and I was able not just to keep still (she is persistent), but also to communicate telepathically that she had to wait, so she desisted.

Then I was interrupted by an AI call from the insurance company wanting a short survey of my last doctor's visit, a clever way to circumvent HIPPA restrictions and trick people into providing confidential medical information. I returned to meditating with just Om (a flavor of Aum, the thought tonality being beyond language). **This brought me into a meditation about privacy and how within the astral dimension one's history is not private.** I understand that this statement contains assumptions, such as that one is observed when entering this realm, but that is the feeling I get when perceiving it open up. Om itself has a penetrating nature, as if one is surprised and reacts with Ohh, then In-Breaths Mmm as if gathering back and re-condensing one's personal energy.

Then memories of a sexual nature arose. From the early encountering of my body as having a sexual nature when I was young to early encounters with women. I was a very conditioned youth to be conservative and not go all the way during my teens, as the sense that I should have a single woman and be married was natural to me, beyond the social convention of the times I grew up in and the 'free love' nonsense. Quantum entanglement is unavoidable in every sexual contact. When I went to California as a wanderer I encountered a culture that seemed to have an invasive nature of being curious about everyone's business. As the astral realm again began to open, I accept my past without shame. I was never mean, cruel, or even manipulative. Failed relationships were learning encounters. Our life history is humbling. Beware of anyone who presents themselves as superior, they are lost in their ego.

As the astral realm became open, I then had the strange vision of a tongue tasting food and of my perception slowly going down a throat, as if eating a bite of food and following it with awareness. It was more than an image and came with sensations of wet texture. It represented a strange transition, almost as a test, as if experiencing this without being embarrassed by the mortal nature of my body or that this set of odd sensations which arose within me without emotional response indicated a successful state of mind to proceed.

I then saw a vast dark pool of water. There was an abstract luminous symbol above the water in the distance and reflecting off the surface. I could not discern the symbol, but it was not a point of light. I like water and went into the water, though it was not wet, nor did a temperature difference enliven my skin as when one jumps into physical water. It was just movement through a dark medium of thick space. I was attracted to go toward the light. The light seemed to form a tunnel around me. This reminded me of looking up at a full moon with a halo and feeling like I was staring down a well at it. I felt no fear, nor any concern that I was dying.

Then briefly a fierce tiger face was right before me, but I remained unemotional, unconcerned, and unafraid. It then changed into a Gorilla, but the creature's eyes conveyed a sadness, as if to pull my heart strings for a species going extinct. I felt deeply for this large and gentle creature with empathy, but at the time was not moved by thoughts of action. It then changed again to an elderly lion. The lion appeared wise and also somewhat tired. **Then I felt the intuited sense of a mighty king who retires knowing all glory in the world is temporary and of no lasting value: time erases everything in form.** The lion was still noble and self-assured. I had a feeling as if it was waiting for me and was at peace with doing so, not judging or hurrying me, just being in its role naturally. Finally I realized I was meditating with the entire four breath mantra. I do not know when I shifted from just Om, but it was a natural process where the mantra becomes a part of me, with its own momentum.

Session 0021:

Hamsa: Out-Breath Hum, In-Breath Sah.

   It took me a while to quiet my thoughts. I found assigning the Out-Breath as Hum needed to be a release, a surrender without effort, which made the Out-Breath longer. Then by really focusing on the thought as the sound and listening to the mantra as I would listen to music, my thoughts greatly diminished. Several times during the session my breath stalled and I went back to the sound and the feeling of release. For most of the session this mantra was natural and effortless. I did not experience the higher Consciousness as a field, but did work with sensing the awareness in my body, from my legs up to my head.
   The first image I received was of a face and it was like mine, but not exactly, then it morphed. I saw many faces, humanoid and all different types of mammal and reptile like forms. The next distinct image was of a cabinet with three shelves. The bottom shelf had many tea/coffee mugs. They were all different sizes, shapes, and colors. I sensed this was my subconscious baggage and needed to have each mug taken out, cleaned, and either kept or given away. In waking life we have a small cabinet with three shelves which requires this task, though the mugs are all clean, it is overcrowded. I then focused on the other shelves and the upper shelf was full of streaming light like the aurora and then a sun rose into the center. Some friends of ours had recently visited Norway and saw the northern lights and those images of the aurora were similar. The impression of the upper shelf was of glorious energy. I wondered about the middle shelf and again saw morphing faces. None of the faces, whether attractive or distorted, curious or fierce, drew any emotional reaction, they just appeared briefly and faded again and again.
   In the next phase I saw a book open with two pages of text. My focus was drawn to the center between the pages, which became pronounced and seemed to vibrate. It became an opening and the sacred symbols of the Pisces Viscera and the Yoni aspect came to mind. The portal to open space was in the center, between the left and right: the center channel of energy. I noted that the humanoid faces I had seen morphing had been all male. This then brought me into awareness of my right and left sides and how they were distinctly different. The right seemed brighter and more pronounced and I understood I needed balance. I energized the dark left by giving it attention so that it had equal presence, without changing its quality of being symbolically darker.

The darkness is the spaceless and timeless from which inspiration, intuition, and creativity emerge: it is the sacred numinous aspect of every living being. I understood that the balancing of the two sides or aspects of my being is required to open the portal. Post meditation I can see that the cabinet's lower shelf is as important as the upper shelf and all aspects of my being and of life need attention and need to be refined. Balancing attention of the left and right in the body is indeed an important teaching to be incorporated into daily life to yield good health.

Session 0022:

SiTa Ram RaMa RaMa: Out-Breath See, In-breath Tah, Out-Breath Ram, In-Breath Silence, Out-Breath Rah, In-Breath Mah, Out-Breath Rah, In-Breath Mah.

    I first started with just RaMa and found Ra to be like a roar of peaceful blessing energy being emitted and projecting forth, while Ma was like a cool liquid filling my body as I breathed in. This is a dualistic balancing of the polarities of the Out-Breath like fire and the In-Breath like water. Since I was just starting the meditation this brought to mind several musical phrases which play between a rising and falling motif. Since this mantra was so balanced, it seemed like a good one for balancing the polarities in the body, but was not going anywhere. I switched briefly to SiTa Ram which had the movement and active energy (Shakti) which the creative feminine Spirit provides the timeless masculine Light of Consciousness (to use the duality language description of the Cosmos as living mystery and Consciousness as receptive life). Male and Female are very symbolic, rather than literal, in this context.

    Once I got the form SiTa Ram RaMa RaMa as four breaths I was on my way through visual astral impressions. The first of which was a translucent bag with a mass of red fuzzy fruit within. This did not represent any earthly fruit I knew, but was highly desirable, and then a voice stated 'I cannot open the bag'. The voice was not mine, but brought up feelings of my inadequacy, which all humans have some of. It also seemed as if it was not time or was just giving me a glimpse. **There is fruit beyond a human's grasp at this time, there is vast potential within the human form waiting to be developed, and having the fortitude to see what power lays dormant is the beginning of healing and seeking true wisdom.**

    The next image was of a vast tapestry laid out as if it were the ground before me. Highlighted and glowing were three icons which I took to be symbols of goddesses, which are themselves symbols of powers (Siddhas) which are available to the self-realized or enlightened person (Jiva-Mukti). The impression on the canvas was of a map, with water bodies and mountain ranges, but I was not able to (or permitted to) see where the map was. Perhaps the three spiritual powers or entities are overseeing that which the tapestry conveys. Perhaps these three powers are aspects of our being waiting to be revealed and embodied to allow manifestation of a superior evolutionary phase of humanity.

The next image is of a dining area which was very upper-class, with a few tables, but which seemed to be someone's private resort. A place to eat, but also meet with friends. There was a counter like table that was right by the windows to the left, with things like a lap top or drawing supplies: I could just feel that this side nook was a solo work area. Outside the windows was an ocean bay, a very beautiful view from slightly above (maybe fifty meters or yards). This was followed by a brief vision of being under water in an ocean current. Nothing is permanent that exists within the currents of time and everything is washed away.

A man is on a stage and the curtain goes down. He has spent all his energy and is just standing there in a daze. Two men come and put an arm around him on either side as trusted friends or assistants. They assist him in walking off the stage. One of them says, "Time for the next act". Humanity is ready for a new paradigm, the current play is in a grand finale and everyone is exhausted. The current way of life is soon to be over as humans wake up to a finer level of reality.

I must add that yesterday we had a large branch come through our picture window. Glass exploded all around me and our dog Rosie, but neither of us was hit by any of it. It reminded me of the culmination to a very clear precognition when a glass exploded and I was unhurt, but a week later a close friend almost died in a car accident when his shattered car window severely cut his neck. Additionally I have been reading about the great flood caused by the Younger Dryas Comet(s) and solar flares (from comets hitting the sun as Earth passed through a dirty region of space), which caused the previous human civilization to perish and even the memory of it to be obscured. Also, when I started, I selected Rama because he represents a protector and in the yesterday window explosion I was protected. The curious thing is I did not associate the various phases of imagery until after the meditation, as I am writing this. Let us hope this is all just past karmic residual and nothing bad happens. No bad event happened following the window exploding from the branch (except costing us money to replace) and no omen was implied. The old maple trees around our house have all died due to extreme shifts in temperature cause by global climate instability and this was the last remaining large old maple tree around our house.

Session 0023:

Sundari: Out-Breath Son-ndah, In-Breath Are-ee or Dar-ee,

 The first note is that thought sound is more flexible than vocal sound which defines the phonemes of language. There was some fluctuation in the exact thought sounds, but using a single breath was natural, as opposed to two breaths with a silent phase on the second, starting in either descending or ascending phase. Once the one breath form was adopted it was so natural as to continue innately and the exact phrasing in mental space transcended language. This invoked a perception of my body within Consciousness which was more sensual than most meditations: My body felt pleasantly physical in astral space.
 The first image was of me as if looking in a mirror. For some reason weeping became a mental buzzword, as song lyrics and poems about weeping arose. The world of humanity is now weeping. So many children are living in abusive and neglected conditions, rather than in nurturing homes. People of all ages are abused by other humans who have lost their soul awareness in the ignorance of believing they are just a temporary material personality. Overall I am not feeling sad and have no focus for weeping personally, but when I see the state of humanity, I see the greed and wars which steal the human potential and keep humanity enslaved in the gravitational well of the Earth. We could be free to explore the stars, but the brightest humans often have a peaceful and benevolent energy and get trodden down by the most deeply illusioned souls. This was not explicitly reasoned thinking as I am stating it, but was as if the overall scent of the global telepathic web was stinking with pain.
 Then a most peculiar thing happened. A small dwarf-like being in colorful clothing ran right below me from the left and I jumped over it to keep it from hitting me, and then it ran off to the right. I inwardly smiled at the bizarre nature of the vision. Of course I was seated in a recliner in an upright position and my feet were on the floor, so the whole jumping impression was completely astral, a vivid dream. That said, there was no sense of the open astral realm or the feeling of being vertical other than for that surprising moment. Tripping on Meditation can be surprising, as can life situations.
 A few times during this meditation I did feel as if my Consciousness was wavering or shaking loose from my body, as if my position was not the sensation of my physical body. My body feels sexual, though not excited in any way, but rather as if my bodily form was naturally

sensual. After feeling both my physical self and my astral dream body I saw a humanoid being with a large head and an elderly appearance very much like a human, but with more of a rounded eye shape and perhaps slightly misaligned features looking into my head, as if gazing into different parts of my personal head space. Then I briefly saw a woman's face with a headband of multicolored thread, with curly, woolly gray hair.

Then I had the sense of looking in a mirror again. I perceived a young boy: I was looking on as an observer, but felt a personal sense as if viewing my past. There was an adult woman who was beautiful and whom the boy was emotionally attached to, getting a last hug and saying, 'I'm going to miss you'. A sad parting. Perhaps some part of my youth hidden in the deep recesses of my subconscious due to the pain of separation. Perhaps a reflection of having just split up the sheep herd, sold off the Ewes and then the ram, and keeping the young wethers, who are feeling alone and missing the elders who they had lived under. Perhaps just a lesson on our attachments and how we must release them to be free and to grow.

This brought me to the problem of the invasion of the rats in our metal barn structure. They had killed and eaten the chipmunks which were enjoyable to have around. I need to kill the rats, but have reservations about killing, however the reassurance arose amid my contemplation stating, 'Kill the demons.' Rats are not demons, just hungry beings who love to breed and so get out of balance. All through Hindu mythology there are demons and the Goddesses and Gods are warriors who kill them to save the good people who cannot defend themselves. I possess a warrior spirit and as sad as it is, I will not fail to defend the children and the good ways. **For some people the spiritual path includes the path of the Warrior, a gentle and peaceful spirit until some demon attacks the meek, helpless souls who are precious.** Spiritual Warriors feed the telepathic web with joy, laughter, and hope for a wonderful and prosperous human destiny. But I offer a word of caution against being judgmental and warn to never harbor hate. Rats are not evil, but need to be controlled or put back in their place. Dictators justify attacking their people and other peoples, but are lost souls needing to be taught a lesson. Some of the most beautiful people are very fragile and delicate and just need space to blossom.

Session 0024:

Durga: In-Breath Der, Out-Breath Ga

    I started with the syllables on the other phases of the breath, but after a very short time, was breathing in Der and breathing out Ga. There was an immediate sensation of a vertical connection of energy within my body, not as moving prana or wind of awareness, but rather as transcendental awareness. I was in a larger space which was comfortable. My third eye was like a horizontal beam of light into the warm darkness. Then in the distance I saw a red door. I sought to move toward the door, but it became diffuse as it expanded due to proximity and the space I was in took on a comforting red glow, as if diffused with a very faint red light.

    I then perceived an image of some tree branches with frozen ice over them, which is something I had seen yesterday and this morning. Beth stated that a large part of Michigan was without power from an ice storm. Then I perceived a fat rocket with a little capsule on top and some white coated technicians below. Beth had also said there was a rocket launch to bring back stranded astronauts aboard the space station, since their return vehicle had been hit by a micro-meteor. Both of these images were the arising from seeds within my recent memory. I also saw some crackers as I had been wondering if they might not be a good treat for the three wether sheep which we kept after selling the four pregnant ewes and the ram. Again this arose from my minds considerations.

    The next image was of ground birds, such as grouse running around under low branches. This is interesting since we only had one grouse show up in the seventeen years we have been here in this rural environment. Only time will tell if the forested ridge which has had the ash trees die will become habitat for such birds. The environment has changed radically in the years we have been here: it is collapsing! Life will persevere, but the fate of our pre-civilized society is at a dangerous crossroad. Humanity needs to heal from its trauma and honor everyone equally and rebalance with the Earth which is the essence of our home. **To be civilized we must find unity as one people while incorporating the richness of all our diversity.**

    When I was coming out of this meditation my lips were tingling intensely and the rest of my body was also tingling. I felt very comfortable and natural with this mantra. There seemed to be a familiarity and easy to using it. I had stated that I would not focus as much on non-repeating images that arise, and yet they tell a story and so I find myself following them in this text. There is a deeper level of time-energy-space and Consciousness which I feel is important, yet is much harder to put into words. I was a bit tired this morning and had the urge to put the back of my recliner down and slip into a morning nap, however I needed to go outside, let the sheep out of the barn, let the goose and ducks out of the protective duck house, collect their eggs, feed the wild birds, and walk our dog around the yard, so I got up and started the day: I returned to typing this soon after the morning chores of a retired man were completed.

Session 0025:

Kali: Out-Breath Ka, In-Breath Li,

It was around 3 in the morning and after waking up to pee, I laid down wide awake. Therefore I started meditating. I soon found myself in the Void. Generally there are the three states, waking consensus reality, dreaming astral reality, and deep sleep which is associated with unconsciousness, but in which I had woken into several times in my life. **The Void is hard to describe, for it is being awake in a deep sleep state: it is not cold, nor warm, but just right; it is not small and confining, nor is it immense and unsettling; and it is not visual to say it is bright or dark.** It is comfortable and yet seemed boring. Occasional thoughts would arise, but I was not mentally lucid, rather I was just breathing Kali. At one point I was aware enough to feel bored and wanted more interaction from the mystery of the Cosmos which I exist within and changed Mantras.

Om BhaGaVaTi DeVi ShakTi ShakTi ShanTi Hum

This is an eight breath mantra which I sometimes use with my Chi Gong movements and so it is very natural and was easy to flow. Like Kali, it was comfortable, but I was still in the Void. I assume that being in conscious awareness in the Void is as restful and rejuvenating as deep sleep. At one point I saw some points of light moving about, but not patterning in symbolic form. This presented the impression of being in a large open space, but this vastness is not the same as that which seems to open in my regular sitting meditation astral space. There is little to generate mental speculation about being in the Void, but there is the feeling that it is embedded in something much greater. In a sense it is like being in a cosmic womb and feeling the presence of the Goddess which is the Cosmos without any distinct qualities to perceive. I feel that so much is concealed from humanity due to our limited senses and our mental paradigm which filters the limited spectrum which we do see.

Session 0026:

Kali: Out-Breath Ka, In-Breath Li,

   Sitting in meditation on Kali many sexual desires arose, some fantasies and some subtle astral sensations. I had very little awareness of my body and the mantra was cycling with my breath so naturally that it put me into a state of watching thoughts arise. The erotic is part of life and everything that arose was a reflection of my heterosexual nature. There was also the component of a presence of a feminine energy, the sacred goddess energy and the beauty of women. There were mostly situational thoughts which had a sexual overtone, but were in themselves not at the stage of sex, rather the presence of desires which are triggered by thoughts or in daily life by some situations, such as seeing my wife's feminine nature and beauty in everyday situations. I cannot recall anything specific from this phase which lasted for a half hour or so. Being human includes having a sexual nature and seeing ourselves truly requires an acceptance of vulnerability.

   The next phase included some astral imagery which was very textually rich. I first perceived a clear glass object embedded in human flesh. It was not specific to any body part, but the contrast between the organic flesh and the shiny glass was astounding. I then saw a cave opening with a light inside it. I was in a dark environment and the cave was in a stone mountain wall and the light within was amorphous, as opposed to a point of light; it had volume and the whole volume had equal brightness and its shining allowed much of the vision of the cave and mountain. Both of these images have a duality: organic and pure mineral in one and light in darkness in the other. Flesh seemed more than the glass and held the glass, while the dark stone held the light. **I can reflect that this is the nature of the Cosmos which is a Sentient Mystery which holds Consciousness within it.** Consciousness has a transparent and also a shining or radiating quality which illuminating my Cosmos.

   The next image was of the top of a salt shaker which morphed into a drain and back into the top of a salt shaker. This implies a filtering and a releasing of wisdom a few grains at a time. It implies the flow of sensory data, which is continual and yet becomes very limited by our mental straining process. We keep some ideas and forget others, but ideas are very dimensionally limited compared to living experience. Reflecting on this brings me to reflect on how in living experience our limited sensory abilities act as the filter and the bits which get through to us are the data from which we create our world, but some of what we currently filter out is what we need to accept in order to enter a more aware state with lucidity. Therefore there are two levels diminishing reality, the limitation of our senses and the symbolizing reflections of our minds. In order for greater awareness to be useful, and for me to process more of my subtle perceptions, there must be the associated spirit to hold focus and will power to maintain attention of the details, otherwise it would just overwhelm and be a blur of data rushing by.

Then I saw the image of a sack of potatoes, which had the quality of a boundary holding multiple objects together. Then it changed to a mass of organic spheres, all bound together by some external pressure, their touching slightly deforming them from idealistic round shapes into joined red and moist organic things. This then changed to a circle surrounded by six circles expanded as a plane of circles, a sort of flower of life, which then changed to three Dimensions as spheres packed together. Although these Euclidean geometry images were not organic, there was a feeling of a message that in the organic world, it is the external container, the boundary and the forces, which give shape to life. **It is more than my skin forming my boundary, it is the pressures of life and the world within which I may define myself and get to know myself.** I reflect (as I write this) that I am both the Consciousness illuminating a filtered bit of the Cosmos and I am also the bit of the Cosmos that is my body and senses. Both must be in interaction for me to be. **My complete body-mind-emotional-astral existence (my active spirit) and my shining Consciousness (my receptive awareness) are equally parts of what I am.**

Session 0027:

Lalita: Out-Breath Lah, In-Breath Lee, Out-Breath Tah, In-Breath, Silence.

 Lalita is 'She who Plays' which sounds like fun, and she has great beauty, but also is the entire play of the Cosmos, continual creation, duality playing out destiny. This was not a fun meditation, but caused to arise many human emotions which we seek to subjugate or ignore, yet they will arise.
 After settling and clearing my mind for a while, the first thing to arise was a memory. I am not going to relate the details here, but just state it was a scene of domestic violence, in this case by the woman against her husband, who did not return her violence, but was in pain. Previously if I recalled the incident it had made me angry, but since I was meditating I did not feel anger or judgment. In this instance I see it was the woman's underlying childhood trauma, combined with her ignorance about how to communicate feelings which motivated such a selfish violent act toward her husband. Often men are even more lacking in communication skills and have suppressed emotions that can erupt as violence. Some mentally unstable people commit suicide, which is self-violence, seeking to end their repressed pain. Most of us carry trauma from various forms of abuse and/or neglect. Middle-school should include therapy for all children so that those who really need help can get it before the responsibilities of adulthood.
 The modern culture has lost some of the natural spiritual nature and this is very disturbing. To fight physically in a relationship is a very sad and degenerated form of living. Call me old fashioned, but there is a loss of the code of nobility, chivalry, and decency; which in a pure form without preconceived rules is a commitment to spontaneous compassionate love. Violence breeds violence and never solves a problem. A mother will fight to protect her children and warriors will fight to protect their community, but these are short term necessities. Communication and negotiation are the art forms which can result in true solutions.
 After returning to the sound of the mantra and the Goddess, the energetic vibrational form of the play or perhaps I should say the drama of the human play, I then encountered competition. It seems in modern times in all the arts there is a sense of competition and striving against others. Thus the arts become clever competition and showmanship, rather than fine creative expression. Indeed in the whole play of life,

people have the competitive energies of 'my will' and 'your will'; seeking dominance and rulership. **Having power over others is a false sense of self-worth and indicates someone is lacking in true self-worth.** It attracts many people in that it is an excuse for not having rulership over one's self and attending to the needed personal growth required to be whole.

It is a complex question in a relationship to balance how much one seeks to impose one's will and desires on another and how much does one accept another person's will and their desires to override one's own. When people fight, it is a sign that they are too immature to communicate and negotiate a balance of their individual paths. The dynamics of people's intent and their will to express their intent is a big part of being in relationship. There is a gender tension in our society which is very unhealthy. It is born from a history of a gross imbalance referred to as 'the patriarchy'. Finding balance and equality of femininity and masculinity, while maintaining their essence, will bring humanity vast healing which is greatly needed in these times of crisis.

I then looked to my future and my desire to plant some trees in the spring. I imagine a peaceful life and the far field where I want to plant the trees becoming a place where humans can share time and enjoy healthy interactions and spiritual discourse for a long time beyond my lifespan. I imagine a small shelter there as a special place to hang out, to play music, and to share with people. Then I consider the turmoil in the world and the cascading collapse of the biosphere and wonder if Lalita, the energy and momentum of the human drama, will allow space for such peace.

From a young age I encountered an establishment of negative controllers who traumatized me as they manifested their selfish schemes. I must admit that another feeling that arises is fear. If I had been treated fairly and respected growing up, who knows what science or art I might have contributed to this society of humanity, but instead I crashed and spent some time as a homeless person. My story is not unique and most children today will not be able to manifest their gifts for the good of all humanity. Humanity needs to change its false understanding of children: the human potential which each of them holds is a precious treasure for the whole of humanity. **Unconditional service to all children equally is that sign of a civilized society.**

I then encountered the presence of one of the Watchers, the Queen Devi, a spiritual and powerful being who is an overlord, who rules with devotion to Lalita, the supreme Goddess or supreme creative sentient energy of the Cosmos. The Queen Devi sees all and knows my whole meditation and life. I felt unworthy and that is another emotion which is put upon children and all people to subjugate their will and mitigate their gifts which could benefit the whole of humanity. No person is unworthy of change and embracing the spiritual path of compassionate love. I felt the need to purify myself, but I am human and such feelings arise whether justified or not. The art of spiritual life is not to stop the arising of feelings, but instead to not allow them to grow within and gain power. I seek to see each feeling clearly and analyze the feeling's source in order to deal with the origin from which it arises. The Queen Devi did not judge me and was not present to cast judgment, even upon seeing all my feeling arise.

I wondered how I could be worthy of the personal presence of such an advanced being for even a momentary flash? What service could I offer her or how might I be useful? Then she showed me a symbolic visual message where half of her face was alien and the other half was of a female human. I felt the message she was sending was not about hybridization of actual physical form, but rather that I can reveal my humanness to her unknowable nature by being myself, vulnerable and revealed. In some ways she knows her oneness with all of life and therefore with humanity and cares about us. As a spiritual overlord in the Cosmos, she has a great responsibility to not impose her will, but to invite us to heal our human nature and become the amazing life form that we have the potential to embody.

As one can see, in meditation many things will arise for one to learn about one's self and become more integrated with what one really is. Ultimately knowing oneself as Consciousness and knowing that the manifesting personality and arising thoughts are temporary reflections from which we may gain perspective and have a better focus to refine our intent brings healing and growth. We do not know the future, and even precognitive glimpses are just telling us about statistically likely outcomes of current paths. The Sacred Mystery, the play of the Cosmos is guided and we need to be spontaneous to makes choices as the changes falling into the path of our life challenge us. Life will redirect us and teach us along this visit to Earth.

Session 0028:

Saha: Out-Breath Sah, In-Breath Ha.

This mantra is said to be the closest to the sound of the breath. After a bit of quieting my mind, I sensed a presence with me. It was non-obtrusive. It seems as if meditation makes one more visible to the Celestial Beings. If this being has a material form, it is very slight and refined, but its world view is focused on the open astral space. I felt the open space around my body as if in a large cavern with light blue walls. The color was subtle, but the feeling of being contained was palpable and comforting.

Next I went through a phase of seeing shakuhachi music, which is written down the right side of the page vertically and proceeds toward the left with each next line of music. I was seeing one line at a time, with the others blurred showing that focus is the key to clarity. I am fluent in reading this notation, but it was distant and I could not transcribe the song. I saw some of the common notes, but it did not seem as if transcribing was the point of the vision. I spend time reading this music and it is getting harder to see as I age and my eyes become weaker. As I continued meditating I saw a more fluid script which I could not read. I was aware that both this and the shakuhachi music were designed to be written by a brush.

I then became aware that there are multiple presences in the open astral space around me as a different type of entity entered my awareness. It seemed more predatory, though the initial being was also a predatory being, as are humans. I had been googling how to use soup bones and some part of me had to consider the reality of the beings who were sacrificed for my food. The initial entity became present again and I felt safe and at peace with my nature. All this occurred in a very brief segment of the meditation.

I again became aware of my body in its totality and also as a boundary floating in open space. As I meditated I felt myself drop briefly out of my form. Contrary to the metal notion of ascending from the top of the head, this was grounded and embraced Earth energy. The exhale is calming, peaceful, and healing. Bouncing right back into my form, my ego mind took the baton and started a dialog about becoming a great cook and pleasing my wife, who has a couple of years until retirement, with a great dinner.

I then went through a phase of slowing my breath and really focusing on the syllables. I perceived a red dot to my right upon the light blue astral cavern walls. I wanted it to be centered, I am not sure why, but it was definitely to my right. I sought to move to it and it expanded like a portal or a tunnel, but as it did so, it faded. I then again focused on the mantra with depth. I next perceived a line to my left in darker blue. It opened like a vertical slit with darkness within. Again I moved toward it and it expanded and faded. I got the idea that in meditation just being is the key, and willfully intending to manipulate the astral images is losing the connection to the mantra.

I again deepened my focus on the mantra and my body as form in the light blue cavern. I then fell out of my body briefly. When this happens my breath almost stops, becoming very faint and thin and the mantra seems more distant from my conscious perception similar to a sound becoming fainter with distance. Re-centering in my bodily form I appreciated the slow and very fine breathing. It gradually returned to normal and my heterosexual male nature engaged in fantasy about the female form, the ultimate attractive aesthetic form within all of manifestation (for me). I can accept the arising of awareness of the sacred feminine Goddesses within our human world view. **Every world view, every paradigm of the Cosmos which exists within mental symbolism, is a mythology, a story, a greatly diminished reflection in symbols.**

I also became aware that these ramblings of my ego included being present with a counterpart who was female at two different sites. There was nothing overtly erotic about being with the feminine counterpart, about being accompanied by a woman or a Goddess. The first instance involved visionary translocation to a Goddess Temple in India where some very spiritual people, male and female of varying ages, were worshiping. It was as if I was appearing to them amid their worship service (Puja). There was incense and flowers and they were enraptured and I got the sense of them perceiving us, the female and I. The second such translocation vision was of appearing to a group of people in the western deserts of the United States who were engaged in modern spiritual practice with some Native American teachers. I took my astral woman companion's hand as we stood before them. The revealing of ourselves in our astral bodies had the feeling of being naked, though I was not visually attuned enough to make out details. In both cases I sensed connection to these groups.

Returning to the mantra and my body floating in the light blue cavern I put forth an intention to summarize all of these experiential perceptions. I then realized I had switched briefly to Sahi (Sah Hee) and there was fire energy in these movements to other groups. Slipping down to connect with the Earth was grounding and cooling, like sweet refreshing water, but these astral journeys were fiery. I returned to Saha and saw a line on the left and a circle on the right. The line was long compared to the diameter of the circle and I understood that the line was Pi and the diameter of the circle was 1. They then transformed into a three dimensional vision: a pillar on the left and a sphere on the right.

The three dimensional expansion indicates that we must somehow conceive of a higher level expansion into dimensionality than 3-D, which cannot be visualized, but which can be felt. Then the two dimensional images overlapped and I saw the vertical line through the circle in the center of my vision. I then saw the three dimensional visions overlapped and conceived of the spatial interaction as electric current surrounded by a magnetic field. This image of the dual nature of electromagnetic energy is the starting point for understanding the manifest Cosmos, as it is an apt simile for male and female energies, God and Goddess, push and pull, the dynamic tension which is involved in all aspects of the grand play of the Cosmos in its unfolding.

Session 0029:

Aham: Out-Breath Ahhh, In-Breath Hum.

 This is a spiritual heart mantra ('I Am') and it has a calming and healing energy. Once I am meditating and several cycles of just the mantra occurs between every arising thought, my body became present. This mantra is a whole body mantra and the process of being aware of all parts of one's body, from feet to head, and this allows one to center and go deeper. The myth that the third eye is just like an eye in one's forehead is dispelled, since all the bodies energy centers must be active for one to slip into the astral dreaming body. One's physical body is present, but gradually one's focus of attention leaves it there while breathing with the mantra on autopilot. The visual images appear before one as if seeing with the eyes, but the body is no longer present.
 The first image is a woman's face, very beautiful and surreal, looking from a position on my right, looking up and toward the left across my center. This was followed by a plate with toast crumbs scattered on it which morphed into a spiral galaxy. I could feel the profound nature of the simile: the stars were like crumbs from a higher point of view. I then saw the sun's surface and a large solar flare, which felt like a reminder that the sun is an active and dynamic body. **Any conception of the Cosmos as static in form is a mental illusion, the Cosmos is spinning with power from the microcosm to the macrocosm, as our breath cycles.**
 Then sinking deeper in meditation I saw a woman's face which was extremely beautiful, neither young, nor old, and of mixed race such that she could not be classified. I was staring at her in awe of the aesthetic beauty. She gave me a look as if to say, 'What are you looking at.'; conveying the meaning without words. I mentally replied, "You are very beautiful. I'm not flirting with you, but I am entranced by your beauty." She moved her body seductively and mentally said, "You can flirt with me if you want." My energy changed, though I had no erotic thoughts, I had to catch my breath. I replied mentally, "You make my heart go pitter-patter."; then my body involuntarily belched. I said in my thoughts, 'Well I guess I failed in that flirtation.' My physical body laughed at this, bringing me out of the astral dream state. Note that in this dream imagery I say the spoken parts were said in my thoughts because there was no specific voice sound accompanying the words. The astral realm is a lucid dreaming state with an energetic power to

reflect one's present life and therefore provide deep learning opportunities.

Back to focus on the mantra and the breath until they went into autopilot again as thoughts became very occasional. I then sensed the Queen Devi. I asked her to show me her form, which I knew was small, frail, and withered by age, yet she did not visually present herself. I asked her again stating that I might have a conditioned reaction, but forgive me for what might arise as I longed to behold her in fullness and grasp her inner beauty. I felt a deep love, free of erotic desire, but stronger than mortal attraction. I longed the hold her hand, to hug her, to be in her presence. I felt unworthy, yet she somehow comforted me. With some very subtle level of feeling of her presence I was satisfied. The bliss of her awareness put me back in my breathing of the mantra and the sense of having a body which was suspended in the space referred to as the void.

Meditating for a while in the void which is not warm or cold, light or dark, or definable other than a sense that I was aware and my dream body was present in vastness undefinable. I then perceived the intersection of the vesica piscis (mandrola), a symbol of the union or connection of opposites represented as two spheres overlapping. It had a warm red energy which pulsated in a sensual way. I took it as a sign that every interaction with Queen Devi was a deep communion of souls and I felt a great satisfaction, rather than an unfulfilled desire.

Session 0030:

IHam: In-Breath Eeee, Out-Breath hoom (like who and moon and ending in mmm).

It took me a long time to settle my mind. Awareness of breathing the mantra and awareness of my body in phases as I calmed into inner peace. Feeling different parts of the body until I am aware of my whole body is a good aid in the beginning phases of meditation and open up the larger space of inner awareness. My first image was of a leather bag, like a wine-skin with a bigger opening that had a plastic screw-on top. I was putting vegetables and stuff in it, sort of like a thick soup, not gross, but not appetizing, and it was all mixing together. I rinsed off the opening where I was putting the mixture. I assume now this represents my mind and all the thoughts arising and being added to a soup of thinking. **Awareness of what we feed our mind can provide discretion in our choices.**

I next saw a solid block of pressed tea. Pressed tea is soaked briefly in hot water before being used. The tea block was there for a while and I wondered what it meant. Reflecting as I write, perhaps it represented stuck thoughts. Our minds are full of assumptions/beliefs which are as if frozen, potentially useful but sitting in an unusable state. I then saw a page of text and then a previous page and then a previous page. **I understood that this meant that my assumptions/beliefs change over time and I need to see how they change and be informed of the implications of their changes.** It also indicates that static ideas must be replaced with fluid growth, not random and chaotic, but fractalizing into greater understanding.

Finally I felt deeper in the mantra and saw many changing faces. I could not identify characteristics other than they were humanoid. They changed between male to female, young and old, and attractive and bizarre. At one point I saw a body, but it was not clear enough to tell if male or female, only that it was young, but somehow not healthy. I did not sense much presence, rather just a diversity of form. Perhaps the faces represented the potential for conscious presence and the sickly youth indicates that many people live life without contemplating the journey. Is the evolution of humanity being stifled by electronics and mindless media pouring into young brains faster than it can be processed with deep thinking?

I saw book shelves full of books on my left, they were taller than a person and under a curved light blue ceiling; however, to the right was a fog of reddish light. The fog was all there was, no ceiling, floor, or objects. The fog seemed to expand slightly and obscure the books. I understood this in the meditation to mean that books contain linear thoughts frozen in time and lack ongoing creativity. This idea is mirrored in the tea block image. All forms of media with fixed narrative are frozen bits of thoughts from the past. One can read endless books, but they do not compare to real experience. I briefly saw a hand with numerous bracelets and understood that these were a tribal way of remembering wisdom in an oral culture and passing along stories which remained vital while keeping an essence.

After being deep in the meditation for a period, I then saw sedimentary layers in a cliff wall which changed into bookshelves proceeding into the distance until they were tiny and faded from view. I understood this to mean they go back in time, representing history in a jaded manner which does not contain the feel or the world view of the historical time period. A person of today reading an ancient text can only see it from their current world view. In contemplation as I write this the example is the Sun and Moon as deities ruling over humanity. Even today as some deep thinkers contemplate Consciousness and hypothesize that the Sun may have some kind of perception, there is no way to return to the world view where they are god and goddess which are personified in stories. Yet we have lost a connection about how deeply they affect our body and consciousness. The cycles of the Cosmos rule over and control all aspects of our nature.

This image was followed by the image of a rocky mountain top with eroded round boulders. Several of them surrounded a deep pit. Peering into it was only blackness. This was followed by a woman's body, her hips swaying, and the insinuation of something desirous. I was contemplating what is the quintessential urge that drives one to seek beyond the bodily urges which give rise to desires and beyond the pain and the fears which give rise to aversions. Some initial urge must precede any action which someone takes. I contemplate what is the urge which impels me to meditate?

Meditation is motivated by the urge to know more about self as a conscious entity, about others, the Cosmos, and the many relationships which entwine and entangle these conceptual concepts. I say conceptual because the entire Cosmos is a vast Mystery and my Consciousness journeying herein is dependent upon the flow of the Mystery, since if there was nothing to be conscious of, how would I be conscious. This is not to imply that my body (a conceptual unit based on sensory data and mental learning) is required, for during most of the meditation I am unaware of my body or the world of waking reality. The symbolism of words is a very limited and presents a limited reflection of the Mystery, therefore such mental ruminations can only go so far. Perhaps the urge to meditate is the attraction of the experience of non-ordinary states of awareness and the interacting with some higher Consciousness. I cannot say that it is the goddess, godhead, or more advanced entities, nor can I say it is an aspect of my own mind's capabilities, but I can say that the experience reflects me and my energetic state in a sentient interaction to provide an opportunity for me to learn and grow.

Session 0031:

Ahha: Out-Breath Ahhh, In-Breath Haah,

I quickly went into the phase where I was aware of my whole body and my attention moved through it and expanded beyond it. I briefly saw an image of fire that was contained in a stone hearth, followed by a net like pattern of energy. I was informed that the weave could be expanded and contracted. This implies that both warp and weft both expand or contract together. Consciousness and the cosmic energy of manifestation are entwined, when Consciousness increases, the dance of the Cosmos holding it increases; likewise they decrease together. **Control the illuminating fire and control the net that filters perception in order to embrace the Cosmos and dance with the events falling from the future into one's life.**

This was an interesting meditation in that I was in the void and fell into dreams twice and woke up from them without remembering their details. Upon returning to the void I returned to being conscious, though not of anything more than breathing the mantra.

Ahha: Out-Breath Ahhh, In-Breath Haah,

A second session in the same day. Again no astral visual energy, this mantra was grounded in the lower Dan Tien, the center of gravity, just below the navel and a bit within (this would be the womb space for a woman). It was body bliss and healing, very grounding. Different than clear void, it was more connected to physical body. It seemed healing. My sense of space around me was more limited, but my boundary was huge, as if my body was vast. There were some moments when something like a field of energy was present around my boundary. This was again a session of bliss, not pleasure, but rejuvenating bliss.

Session 0032:

Om Kali Padme Hum: Out-Breath Ohhh (auh), In-Breath mmm, Out-Breath Kah, In-Breath Lee, Out-Breath Pod, In-Breath Ma, Out-Breath Hoom, In-Breath Silence.

   This variation on the traditional mantra was not what I intended starting out, but was what quickly asserted itself. The usual quieting of mind, body Consciousness, relaxing the body, letting the body become translucent within the energy field took place quickly. A few images arose, such as a handwritten multilevel list and a fractal flower. The instruction arose to remember, as something was between these images. One is linear and one is cyclical. Both logic and creativity are entwined and there is a mode that falls between them.
   I meditated for a while and then the image of a lily pad and flower bobbing on the surface of a pond arose. We do not have Lotus (Padme) flowers in my bio-region but the symbolism works, with roots in the mud and flower in the sun. I sensed the water as a vast pond where the limits were beyond my perception and I was both under the water and above it. It is here that the profound realization occurred: **The rising and falling of the pond of an energy field is what was causing the rising and falling of my breath!** The sensation was extremely complex, but as the energy field wave rose a bit, I breathed in and as the wave fell I exhaled. The vast pond represented some cosmic energy field and my body was immersed in it, but my Consciousness also had a flower above the immersion, a vast open space. This vision faded and returned and faded indicating deep significance.
   I then sensed a very poor mother giving birth on the streets. There was a desire to help, but of course I was just an observer. It was not a graphic image, rather the hopelessness of having nothing for a child and yet bringing the child into the world where it had a low chance of survival. I then saw a very thin, weak old man who was also on the streets with no support and about to die in poverty. In a sense the birth was a wave of the energy field spilling into the manifest aspect of form and the dying man was no longer feeling the waves of energy buoying him up in this realm and would soon slip completely below the surface, losing his garb of a body.
   Then I sensed a Warrior spirit. When I sense violent people attacking the innocent or greedy people stealing or scamming others, I am impelled to imagining retribution. I feel guilty when a thought of violent self-defense arises, yet in the meditation I am pardoned, as if a

necessary action is not evil, for it is not motivated by selfish or other negative intent. **A Warrior's path is a Spiritual path if motivated by compassionate love.**

I then returned to bobbing up and down on the field of energy, riding the waves with breath, which is also time. It is very healing to be conscious of the energy field which is supporting me above the underworld, yet the underworld is a vast part of our beings. We forget the underworld when we are born and conditioned both by the joy of breathing and eating and then by human conditioning, but we can never completely leave it, the vast other side stays within us. At the same time there is a realm above, a bright and clear void filled with a delicious feeling which sometimes flashes into our awareness as a brief intuitive inspiration of divine presence. **Then as I watched my breathing I realized it is also like a bellows, as if gathering a bit of some energy with each in-breath and processing it with each out-breath.** This is deep wisdom which I hope to unravel as I continue this most vital experiential experiment in meditation.

Session 0033:

Om Kali Devi Hum: Out-Breath Ohhh (auh), In-Breath mmm (uMmm), Out-Breath Kah, In-Breath Lee, Out-Breath Dev, In-Breath Vee, Out-Breath Hoom, In-Breath Silence.

In the first try at this I was very body conscious. I felt the energy of the Goddess as very sexual and alluring. My mind kept falling into fantasy. Not the detailed fantasy of a waking state mind, but the deeper visionary fantasy of subtle glimpses of a coquettish woman sending vague and fleeting images which stimulate fantasy. By erotic fantasy I mean nothing as direct as R rated TV, but rather situational fantasy, like being in a coffee house and meeting a woman, only to realize she was an extra-terrestrial, an angel, or a Devi (Goddess) appearing as a human who could read my mind and know my full self as a naked soul. Another example is playing my shakuhachi flute at a small gathering and realizing a Goddess was in attendance disguised as a woman in the audience who could directly connect with the music telepathically which would carry us both through the most intimate knowing of each other. I say erotic because of the strong sexy nature of the 'women' and the allure of the potential which that presents, though being married I am not given to pursue strange women regardless of their presentation. **There is a deep numinous longing which is inherited at birth, the deepest hunger, imparted by the leaving of the unity to have a journey of incarnation.**
Indeed the presence was more than a human could be and was toying with me. Kali is the Goddess of time and also the dark Goddess, representing the vast darkness of our amnesia of the past and also the obscure future. The dark Goddess is a potent and supremely attractive fragrance which is the sacred nectar of immortality (Amrita), which is essence which transcends time and all the energy of light and form which time holds. In a final clear image I saw a hand offer me a small cylindrical clear glass of red wine. Obviously symbolic of an initiation into the divinity which transcends mortality.
In a second session later in the morning I again felt the presence conjured by the mantra, but the mostly obscured faces were just beyond clarity and were of vast diversity. Then after a while I perceived several advanced futuristic machines, some type of high tech and high energy round devices within a room which was filled with high tech gear. This was followed with a tapestry of many colors dancing with floral fractal patterns without a specific fixed image. These seemed to represent

natural imagery as opposed to the high tech cold steel images of the future machines. I was then drawn into the contemplation of the rise and fall of civilizations in a cyclic manner throughout history. The Goddess watches, wishing to dance and play, but humanity is lost in a fantasy of materialism, while the tides of the vast ocean of energy slowly rise and fall over the ages.

Session 0034:

Om Kali Shakti Hum: Out-Breath Ohhh (aum), In-Breath mmm (uMmm), Out-Breath Kah, In-Breath Lee, Out-Breath Shock, In-Breath Tee, Out-Breath Hoom, In-Breath Silence.

    I first perceived a wreath of leaves and inside it was a smaller wreath of leaves and inside it was a smaller wreath; Concentric rings fading into a center vortex which then briefly took on a spiral nature, not limited to two or three dimensions. This is hard to describe in language because the image cannot be visualized in the limited three dimensional form. I then saw line drawings of a male on the right and female on the left, and they became slightly ambiguous as they morphed, indicating dualistic thinking did not contain the mostly similar nature of being a mortal human. I saw a flaming throne, the queen of fire, for time consumes as a fire consumes and only ashes remain. I then saw a fireball shooting from the horizon in what appeared as an ascending arc, but it disintegrated and burnt out, as all life forms will do before the Goddess of Time.
    This was quickly followed by a birds nest with an egg in it; the nest reflecting the fractal leaf wreaths, but holding within something which has the complete code to unfold as a being. Birth and the river of life conquer death in a non-personal way, as if the species is also an organism and the totality of life's river is a being. Then the owl as a symbol of wisdom appeared and I was made aware that the owl is a hunter, a predator with its own needs, as are humans. Wise as we may be, we are bound to our form and its needs and we go forth in life seeking what we need to survive. We need wisdom and should continually hunt for it, for there are many levels of needs and our truest need is to unravel the essence of the mystery of life, as the Goddess of Time gives and takes according to her whims. When one gets to know the Goddess of Time, one learns that as harsh or pleasant as times are, she continually seeks to increase our Consciousness.
    The second phase was where I was suspended just breathing the mantra in an open clear space of awareness. Again I could experience the waves of an energy field which caused my breath to rise and fall. In deep meditation one is aware of the breath and the mantra, but they are effortless and a part of natural being. I was then experiencing the still and timeless nature of the field of my Conscious Essence within which the waves were causing the bobbing of my body rising and falling, breathing in and falling, breathing out. **There is a higher**

dimensionality which can be experientially known, but which words will not adequately describe. The waves which cause my breathing are within the still field of Conscious Essence, they are entwined and the waves are a lower dimensional fluctuation within the higher dimensional still field. To say the field is still is inaccurate, rather it transcends time in some way. When Conscious Essence interacts with the energy which has form as a living being, it remains as it is and yet pulsates with waves in the curvature of space and one of these waves is the breath of a living being.

Session 0035:

AUM Kali Amrita: Out-Breath Auh (as in how), In-Breath Mmm (subtle and fading), Out-Breath Kah, In-Breath Lee, Out-Breath Ammm, In-Breath Ree, Out-Breath Tah, In-Breath Silence.

My first impressions recalled Krishna and Arjuna on the battlefield. Krishna claims to be time and in this way is a masculine version of the Goddess Kali. Time destroys what is and also births what is to be. There is a warrior spirit to life and Amrita, the elixir of immortality from churning spatial geometry was preceded by poison. Arjuna wanted peace, but Krishna urged him to defend all that was descent, civil, and respectful. There is great paradox here, but this is mental speculation and I was urged to focus more clearly and let the mantra teach me.

The waves causing the rising and falling of my breath were the higher dimensional fluctuation in the dual geometry of space, the pendulum of in-breath and out-breath acting like a bellows, gathering some subtle aspect, perhaps the fabric of space itself, and compressing it into life force, which is pushed into everyone's being, everyone's assemblage of form. Thus every breath is a counter measure to entropy and an accumulation of complexity. From birth a child grows its body, but also mind and emotions. The body, mind and emotions continue to develop over one's life, to gain insight and maturity. The mind gains some sort of telepathic remote viewing quality and the emotions which are a higher level gain some empathic feeling to guide the way and discriminate what paths to take and what to avoid. In aging the lower levels of our shell degenerate in time, but something higher may be refined if one has the spirit to do so.

It is true one cannot stop the mind completely, but the idea that in western mantra teachings one should just watch the mind and let it do what it wants is false advice. One should rarefy one's thoughts by focusing increasing awareness on the mantric sound which is following the breath. As one begins to meditate the thoughts are flowing in a continual stream, sometimes intellectual as in the consideration of Krishna and Arjuna, but other times babbling. Then as the meditation deepens one goes for the four breaths of this mantra without a single though arising and this is the beginning of true meditation. Then several rounds pass without a single thought. One can realize in this state that there are higher concepts than intellectual understandings which will arise without thought, words, or sounds, but these are also allowed to pass. Knowing this higher level than the mind's thoughts or mental sounds is a profound step in mantric practice.

One reaches meditation when the mind becomes simple, not stupid, but clear and elegant, insightful, and creatively revelatory. **The mind stops following the next thought and the next and the next like a hungry dog and starts giving epiphanies of true creativity and one's inner feeling changes like a dog wagging its tail happily in just being.** As I was experiencing these insights in my meditation, my dog was sleeping and dreaming and barked in her dream synchronistically at the fact that a simple mind may be elegant rather than stupid and she wagged her tail while dreaming synchronistically when my meditation had the knowledge that a rarefied mind would be clear and creatively insightful. The Goddess of Time is all knowing and the changes falling into the present are always adjusting to one's conscious state.

The next phase of this meditation was a vision of a watering can as used in the garden and the realization that what is gathered in the in-breath in the upper center is slowly poured down the spinal column or central channel (Sushumna). This then fills a pool of elixir in the lower center. Slow and deep breath with the resonance of the mantra thought sound brings the assemblage of one's being into resonance with a specific quality of the geometry of space-time. Breath is a physical manifestation of the waves fluctuating pulsation of the geometry of space-time, and the breath causes the spine to slightly expand and contract and thereby induces a current which then controls the other aspects of one's body and in this way is feeding one's whole being with anti-entropic energy.

The specific resonance of the mantra brings more subtle vibrational resonance and attunes one to very specific cosmic energies. The word Amrita has encoded within it the key to elixir. The Amm is a potentiating vibration and then the cycling of a deep breath ascending as Ree and spilling over to Tah and is the perfect sonic image for gathering elixir from the fabric of pulsating space-time and pouring it slowly to fill the pool of living waters within one's essence. The silence of time and space are completely full of potential for energy and material form. This meditation has clearly demonstrated to me that Sanskrit is the spiritual language which it is purported to be and that sound vibration is the meaning at a higher dimensionality than intellectual thoughts can ever convey.

Session 0036:

Sauh: In-Breath Sah, Out-Breath ooh (au as in how, but riding over the top node between in-breath and out-breath).

    I asserted my will to be without a directive for what to experience. I found myself focusing on being in the presence of, or communicating with, another being on a higher level of communing with them. Devata / Devika, gods, deities, ghosts, guardian angles, extra-terrestrials, and Mother Earth are all ways one can hypothesize about feeling a sentient presence, as well as considering it as one's higher super-conscious self (as opposed to subconscious self which would be instinctual). One might also consider the Cosmos itself as alive and sentient from a non-dual state of oneness with the all. All these types of mental contemplation thin out in meditation and one is left with experiential perceptions and feelings.
    In the meditation I had a vague sense of visual images of faces, but I was not interested in this aspect. I assume that what I see would be colored by my preconceptions. On a deeper level judging someone from their appearance can be very misleading in terms of knowing their character. To truly commune with another being, in meditation or in daily life, one needs to eliminate one's own projections and allow the other being, the person's energy, to flow to you and also your own energy to radiate to the other being / person. Just being in someone's presence is very enlightening and can lead to non-dual experiential experience. In meditation encountering a Devata, a sentient presence, does not require one to mentally cast a set of personality traits or analyze if the presence is one's higher self or external, since in meditation one is the field that experiences as well as one's own body and personality; everything is experienced by one's Consciousness in the same way as the Devata, the sentient presence, is.
    The other thing I came to know in this meditation is that in encountering a Devata one need not put forth desires and expectations on the being. Any time one puts forth demands on another bring, one is visualizing that being in a contracted sense. This can be understood as in communication where spontaneous conversation can flow naturally for a long time in an easy manner. One can even bring up interests without requiring answers or seeking to make a point, but rather simply expressing what one thinks without firm beliefs of it as right or wrong and listening to someone else express a point of view in an equally non-judgmental manner.

Therefore in this meditation I was able to perceive and experience the qualities of presence without judging if it was me or other. In such a non-dual state one can just sense awareness with a deep feeling of knowing. In my masculine nature I tend to sense a complimentary female presence and only after meditation do I make note of this. In meditation a sense of the divine feminine has an energy which naturally attracts me with longing and also fulfills me through its superior nature. I am incited to seek (some abstract thing) and yet know that it is just a play, a game of love, which the presence uses to raise my awareness's vibration. **The Cosmos itself conceals from us endless mysteries and thereby invites us to evolve the perceptual abilities to uncover more, to know her more deeply and fully.** One feels the urge to say 'show me', 'reveal yourself to me', or 'tell me the answer', but at the same time these urges arise, just the dance of perception within the Cosmos, the sacred flow of one's life, is immensely satisfying in the engaged and entwined state.

One can see from the progression in this meditation that meditation acts like a purifier of one's thoughts and emotions. One who can enter deeply into meditation will experience a soul cleansing. There is significant healing in every meditation session, as one gazes into a reflection of their being in the mirror of their thoughts, feelings, and visions. As one knows one's self on a deeper level, one can progress upon a spiritual path and become a more loving humble human being. One's personality can be consciously witnessed and one can realize that at death the ego is completely gone, therefore one will not mistake one's true self for one's temporary personality.

Session 0037:

Lakshmi: Out-Breath Lak, In-Breath Shmee.

   I can philosophize with the sounds according to the tales of the goddess, but yet I seek to see how I encounter Lakshmi in meditation without adding a filter of expectation. If La is Earth and also Moon and water, feminine and soft and Ka is the start of energy, a beginning, while Kala is time, then this is the reversal of time, or perhaps time attracting its desires. This is empowered by the in breath which energizes. My first images were of a woman's beautiful face, morphing to very many different faces and yet beautiful in all their diversity. Then the faces would mature and grow wise, and then the faces became powerful and serious teachers, calm and loving and yet strict and demanding.

Lakshmi Krim: Out-Breath Lak, In-Breath Shmee, Out-Breath Kreem, In-Breath Silence.

   I was soon motivated to add Krim. Kreem is associated with Kali, the goddess or archetype of time, not Shrim which is associated with Lakshmi. I made the change without thinking or knowing the relationships of the sounds, just in meditational deep insight and feeling the urge to add Krim. The fiery aspect of the divine feminine arose, the mother protecting her young ones, the female warrior. From there my meditation turned deeper than astral images and is hard to put into words. Lakshmi is said to bring good fortune and prosperity. What does one desire? Is one attracted to gaining personal power? Is one attracted to gaining youth? Does one seek to open the portal to infinite potential? All these are laughed at by time. The meditation taught me about the value of a equanimous state, neither desiring, nor not desiring, but yet following one's nature. **One may invoke the power of time and the sentient universe to bring about true good fortune according to one's nature, but without qualifying what that would be: invoking to naturally bring about one's most beneficial spiritual progress.**
   There is nothing external which is needed to advance spiritually, to refine and increase one's Consciousness. While Consciousness is inherently beyond time, one has a spirit of intent and a unique personal nature which is seeking to manifest to its highest potential. No material substance can do the work of meditation for you. All abstinence or excessive behaviors make one's progress more difficult. Being at peace

with one's body and its needs frees awareness for higher pursuits. The moderation and balancing of energies so that they all work together in one's life brings harmonic resonance and leads to living a full and satisfying life amid whatever circumstances present themselves.

    Mantra meditation is a key to human life in that it works from inside to the outer and from the future into the present, allowing the potentiation of higher dimensional Consciousness. One's own sentience, the feeling and sensation of one's essence, is a reflection of pure Consciousness, while one's material senses and thoughts provide conditions to learn with. By increasing the clarity and depth of one's sensing of one's essence, one's unique being, one can become satisfied with one's life. Every person has parts of their life which are humble and definite aging is a humbling process. This meditation brought an awareness that amid the troubles of life, one can experience a richness which is transcendental to one's external condition. What is the wealth and prosperity which can remain when one passes through the gateway of death? Meditation teaches one to accept the journey and become more true to one's self, which implies being a more loving person, feeling good about the energy one sends to others in thought, word, and deed.

Session 0038:

Om Shakti Sivaya: Out-Breath Ohhh (auh), In-Breath mmm (subtle and fading to silence), Out-Breath Shak, In-Breath Tee, Out-Breath Shee, In-Breath Vie, Out-Breath Yah, In-Breath Silence.

In the beginning I briefly did Om Namah Sivaya and quickly visualized a triangular wave pattern as if in bands of colors on a cloth. This was quickly followed by an alien in a space suit with a bubble fish bowl clear helmet. Then it was me in the helmet, then a deer, and then several other men, followed finally by many faces, humanoid and animal. I interpret this as we are all in our own bubble, our own environment of our world view. In the meditation I felt like this is humanities issue of communication, that so much separates our souls, from physical through mental and philosophical realms.

Shortly thereafter I found it natural to do the mantra as expressed in this session's header. I was soon in a blissful void state with my body buzzing with energy. My skin seemed electrical and luminous. Time seemed to drift away. I cannot say if I was tired and entered into a deep sleep state consciously, but I maintained the mantra with my breath. I do not have many words, other than it was refreshing and renewing. It was the kind of meditation that was hard to want to wake up from.

On a philosophical note: OM/AUM is the Word and the Way and Yin passive receptivity precedes Yang active creativity. Contrary to the writings of the patriarchy and 1000 CE non-dual Trika doctrine, Shakti, the feminine aspect of the unity, is supreme and the masculine aspect of Consciousness, Shiva, is generated, sustained, and reabsorbed in supreme Shakti. While it is true that any person's total direct perceptions fall within one's perceiving Consciousness, one's total world view is a reflection in one's Consciousness of the Shakti, the Cosmos as a sacred mystery. The Cosmos of quantum truth, entangled in its totality, is beyond the perceptual capabilities of any living being and will always be. Without thinking during meditation, this was the natural and fluid order of the mantra for me. As the three aspects of the Unity, Shakti (the Cosmos of energy in informational geometry), and Shiva (the radiant light of living Consciousness) are really just One, the Unity, or the Way but words fail when discussing the One, since words are by nature dualistic, representing aspects as opposed to the totality and therefore the primary duality is referred to by many names in many traditions.

Session 0039:

Lalita: Out-Breath Lahhh, In-Breath Lee, Out-Breath Tahhh, In-Breath Silence.

    Lalita, the energy of the Cosmos, plays with every conscious entity. The Cosmos as the embodiment of a sentient Goddess teases me and attracts me. Lalita is familiar and yet we do not know her in our waking mind. She is a quality which is supremely rich, yet from the future into our life she drops the attraction of pleasures and the aversions of displeasures. She reveals a little of her presence and then circumstances change and I am left with a quintessential need to know her, to unravel the secrets of the Cosmos of infinite Mystery. Lalita imparts a longing which is embodied in a curiosity to explore uncharted territory and a fascination for her diverse manifestations. **There is this amazing spectrum in all qualities which transcends a dualistic comprehension and embodies a quirky sense of humor which challenges me to observe carefully and accept the extraordinary for the secrets it reveals.**
    Briefly I went into astral visioning and perceived a woman's face, which kept changing in all qualities: its color and hue and its features such as the degree of femininity and various ethnic traits. But it is her laugh that stands out, as if I just caught her playing a joke and she is laughing at her own cleverness and is totally at peace in her seductive nature. She radiates with femininity while at the same time not conforming to any social standards. Lalita is like a refined woman, but with another side that is the wildness of nature and the raw truth of manifest existence. Lalita, the personification of Cosmic personality, is unashamed and plays with mortals like me as if we are her toys, while at the same time she treasures us as her creation and nourishes us within the subtle context of her games of life. Such a deep longing fills my being and even death presents itself as a mystery that taunts me to know it all, while my time slips through the hour glass.
    Then the faces morphed into more advanced humanoid species, beings who would be as a Goddess to a mere mortal like me. Yet embodied in subtle characteristics was the distinctly feminine form and indeed a radiance that was feminine. An androgen insensitive or sexual hormone immune person has a beautiful feminine body because female is the default natural form. These faces of beings which presented themselves in my astral mind eye visions did not have human features and yet were female. Then very powerfully I perceived a super evolved

humanoid, the Queen Devi, who is in communion with a vast web of beings. Many years ago when I first saw her image in meditation and sensed her femininity, she was surprised and departed to contemplate her own nature.

It is amazing that a mere mortal, as I, could surprise a being representing the collective intelligence of a vast telepathic web of beings, yet my groundedness revealed what her subtle and sublime awareness had not focused on in ages. This time I was able to stand before her, unashamed and see her as a woman, for even if her Consciousness swims in the vast interconnected group Consciousness of the Cosmos, she was a being and a woman. Our species are so different that human sexuality was not even a possibility, yet I sensed she had some fascination and feminine need to be attractive in a non-physical way. As a man, I gazed at her and saw her as a woman and I was at peace with her and attracted without lust, but rather with an awe and wonder.

Then the meditation went much deeper. I sensed myself as I was when I was an immature male, a boy child. I sensed a playful woman, one who was sexual and yet not bearing any pedophile urges or thoughts (in this meditational experience). She seemed curious and enjoyed the fact that a part of me was fascinated by her womanly nature. I was aware that when I was an immature boy, I still had heterosexual urges, which were not yet sexual, for one cannot know sexual nature until one experiences it. Yet Lalita, the Cosmos expressed herself to me in such a way that the mystery of all of nature and the mystery of the twinkle in the playful woman's eyes were entwined. Somehow she knew a secret of human nature which I could not grasp, yet it held a promise of some experiential potential that I could not know as a boy.

Now in my meditation I understand that the bliss of meditation is transcendental experientially to material sensual enjoyments. That there are vast astral realms which are accessible through meditation, but that there is a higher level of communion with Lalita, with the Goddess of the secrets of the Cosmos. One can philosophize that I am not interacting with a sentient persona of the Cosmos and that it is all in my mind, but then what concepts would that redefine in my mind as I experientially encounter this amazing creative Cosmos as inherently intelligent?

The nature of human language and the thinking processes are inherently based in communication. Often deep philosophical discourse, both ancient and modern, are presented as dialog. In meditation I can only comprehend the subtle higher dimensionality as interaction with a higher sentience which is beyond my ordinary thinking mind and my ego personality. The sitting with myself is a learning about myself, yet at the same time there is a dynamic quality, as if the Cosmos were presenting a multi-dimensional mirror which subsumed my body, mind, and feelings and which was active in the creative arising of experiential wisdom.

A physical mirror shows a parity reversed image and so a multidimensional mirror of all the levels of my being would inherently present visions and feelings from a unique perspective. Meditation reveals insight into my nature and the primal urge, which is an existential urge, a deep longing to know the secret in the laughing twinkle in the Goddess's eyes. I am an old man and have studied many traditions which all circle around a knowing which cannot be put into words, yet a knowing that can grow within. Meditating for fifty years has offered me experiences which I can only hint at in these words, but the Goddess's eyes continue to sparkle with a radiant enticement to know my nature and the nature of the Cosmos in some deeper way, a promise that there is something more, something spiritual, mystical, sacred, and divine; something that offers supreme bliss and ecstasy, of which I catch the most subtle whiff of a heavenly scent of magical Lalita in the playful dance of the experiences I am offered.

Session 0040:

Kali Ma: Out-Breath Kah, In-Breath Lee, Out-Breath Mah, In-Breath Silence.

The intro was contemplation about time: I had been contemplating the ancient history of humanity, so this continued to arise, even as my thoughts became spread out with breaths of many mantra cycles between them. It appears that thoughts and their arising and flow in our mind influence how conscious of time we are. There are times in meditation when twenty minutes goes by very quickly, as if it was only a few minutes, and other times when Consciousness perceives our breathing as if it is in slow motion.

Kah is a powerful exhale and Lee is an ascending energy inhale, followed by the gentle and grounding exhale of Mah, and this resulted in my meditation of the Earth as my mother and as humanity's mother. The Earth will slam our civilization due to humanity's abusive environmental behavior: therefore, my compassionate nature brought me into a state of trying to reason with mother Earth to find a different solution. I was fully aware that talking to the Earth was like a single brain cell trying to signal my whole human being, yet this was the poetic nature of my internal dialog. Thoughts arose that asked Earth is she could have an environmental catastrophe which drained some inland area and revealed the advanced ice age civilization, which I realize is not accepted by the main stream old school history of humanity, but which I believe existed. If something revealed to humanity a more ancient civilization, perhaps people would understand their unity as a species and the need to avoid the collapse and disappearance of the modern civilization.

In the meditation I was continually sensing catastrophic changes to the Earth's biosphere. If the ocean currents stop, ice age conditions would quickly descend and as glaciers would cover much of North America once again, the tropical coast lines would reveal the ancient culture, but not much of modern civilization would survive such radical change. Stable climate is required to grow food and fodder. I therefore felt compelled by knowing the Power of Time (the Kali of Kala) to seek the Earth's motherly nature and implore her to find a way to heal humanity, such that humanity could become the force of healing. Hard knocks are not required, a new vision of what humanity is and what humanity can be is required to insight a change of heart from the current ruthless and abusive attitude to a more inclusive vision of humans as part of the Earth, acting naturally to embrace a rich future together, which meditation in a group reveals is blissful. **All humans meditating in the now around the Earth are a group force of immense power.**

Eventually my meditation went deeper and I rode the mantra into transcendental space. From there I was very aware of how my perception of time was linked to my breath and also my thinking. I then briefly changed mantra to Ihum (in-breath as long Eeeee sound and out-breath as Hoom). This put me into a heart space of absorbing energy or life force and radiating that living vibration to those in the meditational state and to all of humanity. I entered into a state where the higher sentient presence was perceived. I do not want to label or personify the presence, only that it was beneficent, as a guardian and guide to me as a meditating human entity. I asked that the presence gift the other meditators with needed experiences for their higher good, without embodying a frightening aspect as all powerful Kali, the ruler of fates, sometimes appears. Thus I returned to the mantra Kali Ma.

Time is fierce and yet to be in time is a sacred blessing. I remained centered in my body, in my heart space, and continued to radiate; while also being sensitive and open to receiving. The Earth energy was merging with the higher dimensional energy and filling my being and vibrating through me as a radiance. This was experiential and did not involve thoughts or images of form. The words are not really expressive of the feeling, but then words never capture what we experience except as a dim reflection. There is not ego in offering what one has as a gift to others, nor should one resist in receiving the energy gifts of others.

I am motivated in all exchanges to keep a pure inner state and not impose upon others what I think would be good for them, but allow the higher sentience to invite others to know that which will serve their spiritual growth. **Perhaps the greatest thing we can do for others is to refine ourselves and thereby naturally be present in a life being lived well, with compassion and love.** Kali, the Goddess personifying time, is the mother of all beings and the nurturer of all beings, while also calling all beings to die. Our temporary visit to the dimensions with time and form are a precious gift which we can honor by embracing life fully. When we step out of the ordinary time stream and meditate into a more subtle sense of time, the perspective we gain is invaluable for proceeding in living life in relationship with local and global community, in our everyday interactions and seeking new ways to live in balance with the natural realm of the Earth which we are visiting.

Session 0041:

Sundari: In-Breath Sun, Out-Breath Dar, In-Breath Ree, Out-Breath Silence.

    The first thing I noticed was that I was filling the final silent exhale with Hum (Hoom), a heart mantra. It took some will to keep the final exhale of the two breath pattern open. Once I did, scenes of my past arose, as if in a past life review. Also curious were the instances which arose, not dramatic events, but things like a situation on-line from a month ago, where I thought to write more to a person in an event chat, who really did not understand an immigrant's struggles, but it was off topic. I then got an astral image of a shopping bag with handles filled with rotting vegetables. This image fit the situation, what I hold inside and what others hold inside will perish, but this was also an intro to the teaching being presented.
    The next astral image which presented itself several times was of a black vortex, a swirling hole into the abyss. This varied slightly in quality and at one point I conceived of a relationship to the belly button hole. Then a nipple appeared briefly and I understood the nipple was a positive geometry while the black vortex was the negative geometry of space. I then perceived the threshold of a doorway, as if the boundary of negative and positive curvatures which were in interaction was the way to understand the message.
    At this point the images changed. I started to see the face of the beautiful Goddess which Sundari represents, but it would age or turn ugly. I saw a young pudgy girl, age quickly and then as an old dead body, shrouded in the black of the vortex. **The nature of form is to arise as a positive curvature from within the negative curvature**. The negative curvature, which is somehow related to time, opens up a space which has a tension and energetic potential, which desires to be filled: representing the image of the hole in the medium created by the whirling energy of the black vortex somehow causing a nipple of form to arise. I then saw a cloth flute bag holding a vertical wood flute as if the bag is the boundary of the negative curvature and within it is the human body, the instrument we play our lives upon.
    The hole of the vortex descends and form bounces into existence in the vibrating tension the void left behind as it spirals onward. In the meditation I next perceived a yo-yo because Da-Ri was like one cycle where Dar descends and has power which impels the Ree to ascend. Ree keeps ascending and in most cycles the exhale seems to hardly

happen, but the silence begs a mental sound vibration to fill it. So powerful was the tendency to fill the silence that spontaneously AUM started filling that silence. It is like a recoil of a drop of water hitting a still pond and creating an indentation and this propels the arising as a reaction. All form is like the ripples created by this urge created by the spiraling black vortex creating the void.

As I looked deeper into the vortex I perceived delicate blue light, like electrical scintillation which arose in the potential. Then I saw the black eyes of a Goddess light up in brilliant colors, morphing in fantastic beauty and swirling as if multicolored fire opals were set into motion in a mesmerizing display of beauty. This transitioned as the memory arose of looking into the eyes of another human and perceiving the twinkling light, the invisible and yet palpable glow of another person's essence, which can only be felt when both people are loving and open, vulnerable and at peace. Somehow in those moments of looking deep into someone's eyes when the world of form recedes into the distance and the vortex connects two people's essence. The final image was of walking up to a shear precipice with music having the marching momentum of time. My mind recalled the image of the fool, unable to resist the powerful urge of the potential of the mystery, the future as a vortex sucking one forward with the tension of the silent exhale and the need which is begging to be filled, which all form dances in response to. Naturally the vibration of the Word arises: AUM.

Session 0042:

Aum Kali Amrita: Out-Breath Ahhh, In-Breath Mmmm (subtly), Out-Breath Kah, In-Breath Lee, Out-Breath Ahhmmm, In-Breath Ree, Out-Breath Tah, In-Breath Silence.

The astral field was a combination of red and blue pixels, very fine and pulsating together. Then I moved up a level and the colors were green and yellow. Then images indicated that the green was plant life and the yellow was an overcoat of stars. The red symbolizes fire and the blue symbolizes the water which modulates the fire. Therefore the stars, including the sun and the moon reflecting sunlight modulate the growth of plants and all life on Earth. I was shown that as a person I need to become increasingly body conscious, to be lucid in my body awareness, sensing my total body continually in order to taste the Amrita, the spiritual nectar of great health and immortality.

The two fields exchange energy continually in a pulsating vibratory dance. Therefore, as a person, I should observe all my energy exchanges. This applies to the psychic energy we exchange with other people, often manifesting as emotional radiance which we send out and the emotional radiance of others that touches us through the astral field. Indeed, all the energy we send out into the Cosmos will impact us as it is mirrored back to us in a modified form for teaching our Consciousness to perceive in a more refined manner and our will and intent to learn how to modulate our emotional output. At a lower level the thoughts in our head and our mental output stir up our emotions and therefore we need to be aware of what we are putting out into the Cosmos.

In order to taste the Amrita one must be aware of the emergence of every energy from one's essence. One is tasked with being aware of one's self and then the question was put forth to me, "Why did you come back (incarnate)?" The answer to that will require more meditation, but influences every intent and decision. When one is living for one's essential nature to allow the emergence of one's true energies, then one is offered the Amrita, the sacred nectar which is beyond space and time. One's essence is beyond time and yet it is in the time stream that there are transformations of one's being offering Consciousness the potential of tasting the nectar of life.

Emergence as one's most true self is the goal, beyond vulnerability and resistance, to truly radiate. This requires balancing the two astral fields red with blue and green with yellow. The world will call one into many required activities and yet one must meditate to have the water to modulate the active fire of the longings within. Balanced fire and water both feed the growth, while the heavens provide natural cycles to control the growth and keep the flow of all things in balance and flowing according to an overarching system. The two astral fields intertwine and are always present in every aspect of space and each has its own dual nature which requires balance to be whole for the essence of a person to emerge.

Meditation is experience, direct perception, and the thoughts which arise are experienced, not thought. After one returns to their fully awake state one should contemplate the experience, as one contemplates other experiences in life. Therefore there arises the profound realization that the red and blue fields are the internal dual geometries of my form. Here I do not want to say body and mind, as that is a synthetic duality and the fields are energetically primary. Somehow I contemplate an electric current as red fire and the magnetic field around it as blue interconnecting energy. The green and yellow dual geometry is the external energies outside of my form, out in the world, the entire Cosmos. I contemplate the energies of the heavens and heavenly bodies stirring the geometry of Earth and providing the cycles, the multiple movements of time, which bring forth the fields of life.

In deeper mental contemplation I consider the boundary between my form and the Cosmos, which is not clearly defined, but which is continually exchanging geometry. **The very fabric of space itself is curved in upon itself into standing waves within standing waves and pulses with the exchange between levels. The two curvatures of geometry overlap and vibrate in their interaction and therefore hum with the radiance of Consciousness.** The breath acting like a bellows is using a tension and pressure to move space, informational geometry, from the Cosmos into our form. This is a clear indication that the mantric vibrations of these thought sounds possess a direct correlation to the wisdom they represent: Aum as essence of Consciousness, Kali as Goddess and potency of time, and Amrita, the sacred nectar of life. Contemplating experience provides the data for wisdom.

Session 0043:

Aum Bhagavati Devi Shakti Shanti Shana Hum: Out-Breath Ahhh, In-Breath mmm, Out-Breath Bah, In-Breath Gah, Out-Breath Vah, In-Breath Tee, Out-Breath Deh, In-Breath Vee. Out-Breath Shock, In-Breath Tee, Out-Breath Shawn, In-Breath Tee, Out-Breath Shaw, In-Breath Na, Out-Breath Hoom, In-Breath Silence.

While this might seem long at eight breaths, I have used it along with my Chi Gong and so it is a natural progression for me, a sound series I have internalized. It is a natural flow from Bliss to Ecstasy to Bliss to Ecstasy to Bliss… It is the cycling energy of the Cosmos, rising and falling, brightening and dimming, expanding and then falling in on myself. It is as if I am collapsing into inner space and then emerging and being energized and expanding again.

I briefly got an astral image of a blueish-black silk inside of a suit case followed by a red nipple arising. While there may be innuendo of a sexual nature, I did not have any thoughts at the time and just saw the images appear in my mind's eye and then fade. Then I sensed the pulsing nature of the astral realm, the arising and fading of images and thoughts. Indeed all sensations have this nature of arising to a peak and then dissolving as if a passing bell curve wave. This mantra beautifully expresses the wave of creation, sustenance, dissolution, and infinitely potentiated void which every aspect of the perceived reflects in diminished form. One may mentally conceive of an object as continuing for a duration in space-time, but one is only conscious of it when one has the will and focus to perceive it. All that arises within Consciousness, from physical sensual experience to the experience of thoughts and feelings, follows a wave of initiating, sustaining, and fading away into the infinite void.

When a thought did arise amid the mantra, it followed the same pattern of rising and falling. Thoughts have a trifold manner in that there is the initial impulse, as brief visionary state which encapsulates the concept and which, if it is sustained, is referred to as a mental download, a revelation, or a spark of inspiration and then the thought form symbolized in words. In most cases the impulse and inspiration is immediately followed by thoughts as words in a string which reflects the meaning intended in the initiating phase. Finally there is the end of the word stream which has a subtle quality of an urge for the next sentence or thought stream to follow. In deep meditation this urge is left in its subtle form, as if a fading ripple and no additional thoughts follow, lest one slip out of meditation and into regular mental activity. In meditation one observes that thoughts arise, progress, and pass as a wave. One does not ignore them, for they may hold profound meaning as a reflection of either one's self or of the inherent meaning in the thought sound of the mantra, nor does one engage the thought to fall into an ongoing river of mental speculation. Meditation is not contemplation, it is a free and pure state of being.

To return to the only two images I perceived in a spontaneous manner: The colors of red and blue were employed but the Cosmos into my meditations and in an extremely wise and clever manner with no formulation by my conscious thinking process. The inside of the suitcase was like the inside of a body, a negatively curved space with a longing potential to be filled, itself cold with the emptiness of pure Consciousness, yet able to hold the blue-black silk of a mysterious natural potential. The arising of the red nipple has the shape of the positive curvature of space, of expanding in round curvature, warm and sensual, as if a physical bellows expanding to pull in the negative curvature of Consciousness and then pushing out to infuse Consciousness with the primordial urge of embodied form. While this may be interpreted to hold sexual connotation, if one contemplates deeper it is the pulsation of Consciousness within the mystery of the Cosmos that is implied, yet sexual longing mirrors the deeper and more profound yearning of the essence of our beings to fill an abstract sense of emptiness.

When meditation frees my Consciousness, there is only the many pulsations of experience and they all follow the pattern of bliss as the base state of the void intensifying into the ecstasy of conscious sensual experience in the now and the releasing back into bliss of the void. **The dual nature of the geometry of space, the void which has infinite potential, as the incredible urge of the future and the manifesting Cosmos of one's experience slipping into the past with echoes into the present boundary as momentum are seen in meditation.** The boundaries of a living form are continually exchanging energies from within to without and from without to within. The boundary of a living being can be poetically described as translucent and possessing its own color, while also having the color of the environment, where color refers to qualities and energies on all levels, such as physical, mental, emotional, and astral.

The individual as a manifest being is entwined with the Cosmos and the pulsations within Consciousness, the most primary essence of one's living being, are also entwined with the Cosmos. The many flows of time as natural cycles and also bodily rhythms are synthesized by

Consciousness into the unified sense of a now which is deeply affected by the changes falling from the future and dissolving into the past. One's situations and multifaceted environment colors one's conscious perceptions and in meditation one releases conditioned influences and there arises naturally the spontaneous experiences within one's Consciousness to learn from. **These meditation experiences are a combination of the deep personal past echoing into the present and the Cosmos, which is the manifestation of the informational geometric tapestry of all things, including the interwoven human form, speaking symbolically with ever new perceptions for lucid Consciousness to process for transformative growth.**

Session 0044:

Tara: Out-Breath Tah(r), In-Breath Rah.

Tara is the protector energy and in story she was acting as a mother and saved Consciousness from the poison of ego which arises as time churns the oceans of humanity and she incites the intent for treasure which is immortal. The mantra brought awareness of the illusion which humanity gets fooled by which is that any material form can resist dissolution or that anything is static. The only thing that remains beyond time is the quality of the feeling of a life well lived, a life of compassionate love. This mantra was mostly emotional energy, it was deep feelings, and the motherly quality to protect and nurture life and the insight was felt beyond intellectual philosophical ideology.

The first set of feelings to arise astrally was the powerful impression of the Earth and the need to support the healing of the environment. Without the Earth being healthy, humanity as a species will fade as all species eventually do. The Earth as a living being and brings forth successive layers of more refined Consciousness. Humanity is a very fine wave with much more potential than is currently being expressed. Indeed the potential of humanity is vast and as yet unmanifest could be our future if we honor the Earth. **The Earth will heal humanity when humanity collectively loses the ego and admits that we have serious problems as a species and we need to mature in order for us to succeed in expressing our potential, rather than failing as a species by failing each other. Either we are one people on one planet or time erases us.**

The next set of feelings was about protecting children from the perpetrators of abuse and violence and this also applies to all humans who are innocent and helpless. These feelings jumped to the need to protect all people from the violence and abuse of the more powerful ego filled lost souls. This applies to people in war torn areas, but especially children who are in developmental stages of life and will be scared for life, sometimes even without clear memories of the abuse they have suffered and yet having to live with triggers which bring forth feelings such that their lives are then never quite right. Everyone has some trauma in life to work through, but severely traumatized people are dysfunctional and yet it is possible to face the challenges they have endured and to become very functional, as well as kind and gentle people with healing to share for others.

This mantra is the Warrior spirit to protect the Earth. In my personal life we just had a two day power outage and so I feel the need to maintain civilization because if it crashes, those who survive, especially the children will be severely traumatized and the tales they pass on will be as those we have inherited, fierce and savage. Humanity has a subconscious sense of sudden disaster from the Younger Dryas catastrophe and the flood which mimics the trauma of an abused child. Humanity has a great need for healing and ending war, along with all sense that anyone is more important than anyone else. Every living human being is on a journey to refine their compassionate love. The vulnerable and defenseless need protection and a sacred living space to grow and offer their gifts. Without their gifts humanity is struggling and time is swift to cut off and discard species which do not change with the times.

This mantra is the Warrior spirit to protect the children. There are many parents who want to put their own desires before the needs of their children. When one brings a child into the world, one may consider the child a temple of divinity and therefore one is obligated to serve that child's needs physically, mentally, and emotionally: a true parent becomes a servant (which can be very humbling). One has a moral responsibility to the child. One's desires are different than one's needs and one must take care of themselves to serve the child in a holistic manner; which does not include spoiling the child, even though it takes less personal effort to pacify the child by allowing them to indulge and is an easy path. Children have a primary need for the attention of their caregivers, meaning full awareness interaction. Everything one does in any relationship has a lasting impact and children are completely open, therefore one must employ one's highest sense of virtue and humble human compassionate love in relating to children.

Session 0045:

Om Namah Shivaya: Out-Breath Aummm, In-Breath mmm into silence, Out-Breath Nah, In-Breath Mah, Out-Breath Shee, In-Breath Vie, Out-Breath Ahhhh, In-Breath Silence.

    The first phase, as my mental activity was becoming more rarefied, I started to perceive the level of mind which precedes thoughts arising. **I did the four breath mantra with no thoughts and then after a round or a few there would arise the thought impulse, the condensed form of the mental urge, which holds all the information of a thought, but without words, without the complete sentence that would be required to think the meaning.** This is profound since it represents the higher form of mental power which is less manifest, but holds the pure essence of what a sentence or a few words hold. I let these also pass and be rarefied such that the breath and mantra assume an automated quality, poetically 'a life of their own'. The ancient meditation texts describe both these phenomena, but only in advanced meditation does one become clearly aware of them.

    Then I entered into the astral or dream vision state, I perceived a red dimple, but it was arising from the inside of a blue sphere. **Therefore the positive curvature arises inside the negative curvature.** The negative curvature expands inner space and then there is a tension of increasing potential within which positive curved form arises. This was followed by a woman's green face, as if she was the Earth energy and she was looking up and her face was bathed in yellow sunlight and she was smiling at the pleasure of absorbing the warm and pleasant energy. This green and yellow vision represented the outer reality while the red-blue represented my inner reality, my being of body, mind, and emotions.

    I briefly wondered why these colors, then thought of orange and could see orange and thought of brown and could see brown, but quickly realized that imagining and manifesting inner vision according to my will was not meditation and had no power for learning the essential truth. I cannot say that what arises naturally has an external source nor that it is a facet of my deeper sentience, only that when I willful imagine things, they are of no value. I have seen many people doing guided meditations and have people imagine this and that, but unless those hypnotic sessions open up to allow for the spontaneous and unguided natural creativity to arise, they will not profit the person doing them. What arises without any willful guidance (from one's thoughts or an external guide) presents a true reflection of one's quest in life, with the answers to one's innermost passion to know the essence which is beyond all one's desires. The spontaneous arising is at a higher level than thought sentences and accompanies the visionary aspect of one's lucid astral journey in meditation.

The next image was of a huge sphere. The thought of a Buckminsterfullerene (C60) arose in my thought at an initial impression level, but was quickly confirmed as not relevant by the feeling of the thought. The sphere was to the left of my vision and was green, but was a lattice in the form of geometric polygons and in the holes was yellow structure permeating it, also in geometric lattice form. Many inner layers were felt or implied implicitly in the layer of wisdom which was deeper than the visual or my analysis. I also sensed the blue was the inside of the lattice ribs with red nodes of form arising within them. Thus the entire structure was a complex model of the Cosmos.

This was followed by a blue male face which was serene and exuded a sense of being: exuding what he was in fullness and the manifesting of the power of his nature. He was looking up as the initial green female face was, but was not illuminated by yellow sunshine, but rather was peering into the void, the dark infinite potential. Potential is embodied as a sacred feminine quality of the void, the womb of the Cosmos filled with everything and the sacred masculine quality radiates the light of Consciousness into her dark mysterious infinity. To use the gender metaphor is very poetic and an ancient way of engaging those who do not really understand that we are discussing the interaction of space and time. The deepest wisdom will be found in understanding this primary duality and transcending it into unity, but the use of words or astral images can only symbolically give one a hint and the true wisdom must be at the finest edge of the impulse of pure knowing before images or words are formed.

Session 0046:

SaHam: In-Breath Saahh, Out-Breath Hum (not Ham or Hoom).

    Saham is a natural sound of breath, therefore it is a mantra of being. The first image I got was of a man with a beard. It could be me, but in the meditation it was just symbolic of divine masculine energy. **The sacred feminine is sterile and barren without the divine masculine. The divine masculine is lost and purposeless without the sacred feminine.** This expresses the fact that the Cosmos without life is sterile and barren, while Consciousness without the dancing Cosmos is in a void of deep sleep and is unconscious and therefore non-existent. It is the sacred feminine, the dancing Cosmos, which gives birth to the divine masculine, Consciousness, nourishes it, and reabsorbs it.

    The next image was of a table with stuff on it, at least some of which was spiritual paraphernalia, but it was not all orderly. As stated in the introduction, one needs nothing external to meditate, meditation is connecting to ones deepest essence which is beyond masculine or feminine. Each person's mind is like a table with lots of stuff filling it and it is not all orderly. Meditation is an art to sort out what is within. It is where we see what arises which is our unique reflection, and then we can decode what belongs, what needs to be filed away, and what can be discarded. One may dabble in many practices, but in order for one to mature, there must be a decision that a specific practice is in harmony with one's nature. As mathematics is the queen of all sciences, the art of meditation is the supreme queen of all arts. **One must tap one's receptivity and accept inspirational grace in order to be a truly creative artist, and meditation is the foundation of receptivity which sees through the clutter on the table of the mind.**

    Space then opened out and was particularly vast to the left and right. As a human we are horizontal beings, that is our spatial navigational conditioning. I had the feeling that before me was the center of a torus of space, that the inside of a torus exemplified the negative curvature which reconnects with itself out of view. Thus left and right extend in curved space until they are connected. This would apply to forward and backward, as well as up and down, all simultaneously connecting within the higher dimensionality within which our three spatial dimensions are embedded. Note that the three senses of direction are not accurate in higher dimensional space, every direction is looping spatially and spiraling with time, This image was followed by a hieroglyphic image of squares, as a mosaic of tiles, which is a visual representation of the human conditioning into linear Cartesian coordinate thinking, rather than spherical and overlapping space. Spatial dimensionality is nestled with layers within layers.

Finally I saw an image of a body as a black outline with lines of measuring sticks about it and as I focused it was female, which is a default orientation. It is the negative curvature of space itself, which forms all the archetypal bodies that exist in nature. Bodies are positive curvature and yet they are also permeated with negative curvature which unfolds them and manifests as growth and aging. **Time is a concept of the negative curvature of dimensionality at a higher level than our three dimensional conditioning.** Time is continual transformation, the unfolding and refolding of the weaving of space.

Session 0047:

Aum Lalita: Out-Breath Ahhhm, In-Breath mmm (a subtle carry over), Out-Breath Lah, In-Breath Lee, Out-Breath Tah, In-Breath Silence.

    I shuffled through mantras and this one stuck and gained momentum. My body was amorphous and yet there was bliss without form. Occasionally I felt my hands existing with form, but vibrating with pleasant energy. There was no specific focus and yet a type of buzzing throughout my indistinct body. There was a thunderstorm and sometimes heavy rain going on outside the house and yet I felt peaceful and at ease.

    I sensed the presence of the Queen Devi and sought a teaching. Rather than controlling the imagery, I simply requested guidance and teaching. Then I sensed another woman, I sensed her laugh and some quirk in her voice. There is nothing describable here. She had a specific energy and a deep familiarity. I was aware of the Blue Devi, the wild one, and as the wind caused howling sounds I heard her howling. The Queen Devi warned me that she was crazy and dangerous, yet somehow the Queen Devi controlled her to an extent and could offer me to her. I am not seeking to be a sacrifice and yet there are times when she is the sweetest woman, sensual and exotic, willing to lead me in a dance.

    Wild Blue Devi reminded me of a human woman I used to sometimes dream about, but whom I did not know in my day to day life. This was profound, as she was such a part of my life for a while and then life went on and I stopped dreaming of her. There was also a blue aura about her and a powerful and unabashed sexuality to her. She was also a creature of the night, hidden in the shadow of dreams and yet having some real nature. I wondered if she was dead or alive somewhere upon the Earth or if she was ever a living human?

    Coming out of meditation she is still like a memory which is suppressed, but occasionally presents a faint inkling of having been. Meditation in this session was able to bring up something of my past, even if just a number of energetic dreams. Some part of my past was making itself known again, reminding me of something both richly pleasant and yet also painful. **Meditation is the most potent tool for healing the past, for retrieving one's spirit from the past and returning one to wholeness in the present.** In this case I do not know what these feelings are or if they are grounded in physical reality, but psychologically there is release of that part of me which was stuck in the past.

Session 0048:

Soma: Out-Breath So, In-Breath Mah; Occasional SoHam: Out-Breath So, In-Breath Hum; occasional Sri Hum: Out-Breath Shree, In-Breath Hoom.

Soma is the lunar nectar of healing, rejuvenation, and wholeness. The overall energy was very mellow and relaxing. Early on I got an image of the full moon with an overlay of stars upon it. This was like a diagram image: no stars were seen in front of the moon, but lines of stars made constellations and a dragon image was prominent. The meaning was to convey a celestial energy being focused and directed to the Earth by the Moon. I felt an impulse to focus energy with dedication to the group of humans meditating around the world, where Soma is the essence of seeking union (Yoga).

I used Soham to reground and stay aware since I kept falling into a blissful stupor. Sometimes thoughts would arise about daily life. I focused an intent to provide the meditators of humanity with energy. I learned long ago that I was an energy or intensity generator, rather than a focus person who would apply the energy to a specific task. Then I was hit with the guilt of ego, like here are a group of meditators and who am I to be one to send energy. Then I realized everyone has special gifts and one should offer what one has. This is not ego nor a desire to be superior to any of the others. Our society will provide many memes which are designed to diminish a person, rather than empower them. This realization is a healing I need to experience repeatedly since in childhood I was continually beaten down.

Finally in reference to Sri Hum: the Goddess Shri (Shree) represents the supreme energy of the Cosmos. Hum (Hoom) is an inducement of power. This is a mantra for sending powerful energy to others, but the energy is not mine. It is me opening up the cosmic energy grid and allowing the energy to flow through me. I saw Goddess statues falling over and into the ground, for the Goddess is also the recycler of energy. This was a clear sign that the Goddess does not need human images to be empowered in people's lives. No one can erase the Goddess as patriarchal societies attempted to do. The Goddess is the giver of life and the entire creative Cosmos.

As the Moon may channel specific celestial energies from the stars, we may channel the cosmic energy and share its healing potential. **Allowing ourselves to surrender to the greater ways of the Cosmos and be filled with the healing of a good life, a life being lived with**

compassionate love, is a spiritual life. Offering flowers and incense to statues is not spiritual practice. One may say it helps one to focus, but close your eyes and meditate on the Goddess' name with your breath and you are going to actually be experiencing the living vibrations offering teachings. This meditation reaffirmed that I can offer my unique gifts of power without it being egotistical.

Soma is very much an extremely powerful set of vibrations. Soham is a very famous powerful mantra and the inhale is matched in Soma. The exhale Ma is the generic term for mother and a key mantric exhale. A baby lamb calls out with 'Ma' to its mother sheep (this is very instructive about the primal nature of some sounds). Ma is the symbol for the protective and nurturing energy of a mother. So is the act of receiving breath and therefore receiving celestial energy. Soma is the mantra of getting nourishing teachings from the Cosmos. It has a quality of providing satisfaction and completeness.

Session 0049:

Bhairavi: In-Breath Bhie (as in Buy but with the h added), Out-Breath Rav, In-Breath Vee, Out-Breath Silence.

   I was very tired, having been up very early. I quickly settled into a blissful state and felt energy moving through my body, then quickly entered into larger space and fell asleep. **There is a concept known as the file drawer data, where people reporting on some subjects, but only write reports about successes and file away the failed attempts giving the impression of always being successful, but I am reporting honestly.** While I am very skilled at meditation, my body needed a nap and thus that is what the meditation brought me.
   I will note that I only sat for the type of meditation I am writing about when I felt energetically called to do so. I do many other meditations which are just luminous bliss which has a healing and rejuvenation quality. Sometimes I wake up at three in the morning and meditate. Often when I perceive astral images I let them slip away like dreams. This record of meditations is of formal sitting with a notebook and when images arise, coming out of the deep state to jot down notes so that I can share the wonders and joy of mantra meditation.

Session 0050:

Bhairavi: In-Breath Bhie, Out-Breath Rav, In-Breath Vee, Out-Breath Silence.

Bhairavi is the Goddess representing the Cosmos who teasingly asks Shiva (who is Consciousness itself) what is the answer; a story personifying the Cosmos presenting itself as dualistic Consciousness with a burning desire to find meaning. My vision was first of the Queen Devi and then there was a sense that there was a mass mailing and some letters were left on the porch and did not go out. The interpretation I feel is that many in humanity are no longer connected to the Cosmos, to nature, and the miracle of Earth, and they are not getting the cosmos's letters of invitation to be a spiritual seeker, to unraveling the science of human nature, and find meaning in their life. **The Watcher Queen Devi then presented the words, and words are rare from the sentient visitors to meditation, "I cannot govern." (meaning rule over). This implies that the most important aspect of human growth is freedom, that true learning must be experiential, we must learn our own lessons in life to fully embody the truth of the meaning of life.** Bhairavi laughs and says, 'Or is it all just me!', the dance of the Goddess.

I then encountered the inverted isosceles triangle, Bhairavi's symbol (representing the energetic Cosmos) followed by the pointing up isosceles triangle of Shiva (representing Consciousness), both with a trinary nature joined in a six pointed star, representing active engagement in union. Then I was instructed that such symbolic diagrams and indeed even words cannot reach the mystery. One's Consciousness must actively dance in sensual-perceptual love with the Cosmos with every life experience. One must be completely present and totally engaged with life in a manner that transcends mental overlay in order to feel the blessings.

Then I digressed into thinking about our dog and goose almost getting into a fight earlier today. There was a fence separating them, but the dumb goose teases the dog and would stick her beak through the fence. The dog once bit the beak and cracked it, but it healed, though it could have been fatal if I had not freed the goose from the dog who had enough of the gooses teasing. This time I pulled the dog back, but then the dog was leashed and was pulling and growling while the goose being fenced kept honking and jutting its beak through the fence and these were the images I was left with. The natural Cosmos has a fierce aspect and Shiva has ego, boasting himself with countless spiritual texts and methods, but Bhairavi is the supreme Cosmos channeling life and offering her supreme gifts to humble and teach the Conscious spirits of all beings.

I considered the many ways I am limited. My human form, especially as I age, has many limitations. I am constrained by the form I am visiting the Cosmos in, not just physically, but on all levels: every human has many limitations. Even my needs are a form of constraint for I must seek to satisfy the body's requirements, and also the mind's need for data to figure things out with, and of course my emotional needs are required for the body and mind to be balanced and functional.

Then the Cosmos presented me with additional words, "So now I just need to figure out what I'm doing [with my life]." This involves dealing with the human world and also the natural aspects of life as a human on Earth. There is a need to clear out mental clutter and to be present in experience, to live daily life lucidly. I am in my senior years and have enough materially to live within humble constraints without worry and I know that nothing accumulated can pass through death's door with me. I read books and learn new word patterns, thought structures, or world views as symbolic maps of the Cosmos for guidance, but ideas will not go with me through death's portal.

There is something about living with transparent integrity and sharing one's gifts which is satisfying (and so I share these tales), yet there remains a longing, an unfulfilled mystery yearning, the whisper of Bhairavi directly to my Consciousness asking what is the ultimate meaning, beyond the mental meanings, what is the supreme and timeless nature of my essence. The Watcher Devi accompanies me from the shadows, some sentience unseen, but for all her advances into super-Consciousness, she still feels the yearning and also lives the mortal journey, even if it is at a sublime level. **What does a humble man like me mean to her transcendental self to be worthy to garner even momentary fragments of her grace, her time and attention?** I do not know, but the sentient presence, whether a being, the Cosmos manifesting, or my own imagination teaches me and I am grateful and feel blessed to receive.

Session 0051:

Hallelujah: Out-Breath Hah, In-Breath Leh (vowel like 'i' in it), Out-Breath Lou , In-Breath Yah.

Note that the 3 primary vowels a, i, u, followed by Ya the seed sound of the ether makes this a very powerful mantra, most likely from an oral tradition where it was so powerful it was never written. Written text and language is a very small part of humanity's spiritual history. My first reception was a visual of a woman's head and her hair was up and around her head as if a flat headdress, with beads around the head part. There was an Egyptian feel to the image. I assume the most essential Sanskrit sacred vibrations were shared orally around the world as teachers left India when later cultures like Egypt arose.

Next I perceived a field of blue energy and it was vibrating and a red mound arose from the center and there was pulsation between the red and blue. Then there was the green and yellow overlay and then in this combination space opened up. The other dimensional space had a quality of also possessing three dimensions, while not being the as limiting or confining as physical dimensions. Then a deep corridor opened before me, a rectangular walkway descending on a twenty degree slant toward an opening which seemed to contain more light and also trees and life as if a wooded meadow. I traveled down the squarish tunnel, but did not reach the end. My body was moving as if walking in a lucid dream, but realizing it snapped me back to my sitting form.

Then I went back into the open dimension and it was like I was in a temple of stone with some natural light filtering in. It was a shadowy space, but there were columns and other large stone objects which I could not make out clearly. This is significant because the open dimension has characteristics and features to be explored. I saw an opening as if two doors with a lattice and bright sun outside coming in. Again as I started to move and my movement in that space startled me and I was back in my body breathing the Mantra. **Interesting that, similar to lucid dreaming, the awareness of being solidly in astral space causes a visceral reaction and pulls one back.**

At this point I switched to the mantra Sauh, the spiritual heart mantra. This was a time of consciously sharing energy, of transmitting energy for others to feel and resonate with, to get to a deeper level. The mantra Sauh is a very sensual mantra, but the energy I was sending had a pure quality so that I intentionally did not change anyone's meditative orientation and yet all present in humanity's collective telepathic web could use the energy. I opened the temple again and felt a deep sense of a sacred space. When I moved to be more aware, it was a little like being out of my body and in my lucid dreaming body and I bounced back into my form. **I returned to Hallelujah and continued to share sacred energy by assuming a state of peaceful communion, sitting together in the telepathic web with inner peace which contained the intensity of Consciousness, yet remained serene.**

Session 0052:

Hrim Krim Shrim: In-Breath Hreem, Out-Breath mmm, In-Breath Kreem, Out-Breath mmm, In-Breath Shreem, Out-Breath mmm.

    I started with a different set of seed mantras, but after some options, settled naturally into this set. The meditation began with sensing energy moving between the lower Dan Tien and the Upper Dan Tien through the heart Hridayam. Then I briefly saw a silver chain with a clasp in the middle. Since the silver cord symbolically connects the physical body to the astral dream body, I felt the representation was a reference to this and the clasp in the middle implied that it could be undone and the key to opening it was the heart space. The silver chord is also a reference to one's sexual partner who's silver cord is twisted around one's own silver cord.

    Then I saw the word 'OPEN' in broad sign like letters. In the meditation I did not relate to the clasp above, but now writing this it does seem that some chain binding me is to be released. I felt the presence of a Queen Devi, one of the telepathic and psychic interconnected transcendental beings. I felt the presence remaining for a while and then saw another word, perhaps 'Bhairavi', but I could not be sure, as it was not clear enough. I then saw a tally sheet, like an excel document with a number column, then two text columns, then a decimal column, perhaps money. I cannot say what this was to mean to me while meditating. Bhairavi is the sentience of the totality of the Cosmos and is personally and intimately aware of every being. **The Queen lingering for more than a brief second is a great honor. She is super-conscious and even a brief glance is a long time in her perspective.** I understand we are all analyzed and contemplated by higher beings. Judged might have wrong connotations, for we are loved and yet this is not referring to our constructed ego personalities, but rather the quality of our true self essence and the feeling we radiate into the Cosmos. **The Queen Devi is in communion with the Cosmos and serves the sacred Way.**

    I was moved then to open my hands which had been folded on my lap, as if open to receive. I must say I presented the Queen with the invitation to communicate with me. Can you be vulnerable enough to be present in the physical realm? Can I touch your material hand? Can you embrace me with a hug? My own sense of vulnerability was much less than my curiosity, though I received no answer, the Watcher seemed to hide more in the background. I sense that we are each in relationship with the Cosmos from a unique perspective and we must attune our being and find our way which is in harmony with the sacred Way.

I then saw an image of a woman's face in the center of a rainbow, where the rainbow was her hair. She was brown and her body was only briefly present for a quick glimpse and seemed almost like a wooden statue with a flowing dress. The image presented would make a beautiful art print and perhaps I will try to create it. **Perhaps this is my answer, that the Queen Devi is somehow a cosmic aspect of the living Earth and not humanoid, but only appears as such in my dreaming in an attempt to be present in my Consciousness.** She, the Queen, seems to be fascinated with my meditation sessions, as if meditation is bridging some gap which humanity needs to cross in order to communicate and be taught. Meditation is an ancient art and the fact that most have lost and is a key component of humanity's very sad step back into being savages engaged in wars.

Session 0053:

Hrim Lim S'rim: In-Breath Hreem, Out-Breath mmm as a subtle residue, In-Breath Leem, Out-Breath mmm as a subtle residue, In-Breath Shreem, Out-Breath mmm as a subtle residue.

    Traditionally the mantric seed symbol is Krim, because k is the first Sanskrit consonant, but as a 'thought word' Leem seemed much smother. In this mantra you have fire before and after the strong sense of water in Lim. This would be similar to the Fire Trigram, but since the water was so strong, it had a balanced nature.
    I went into this meditation with intent to focus on the presence I refer to as Queen Devi. Indeed I had the sense of presence and that presence was ever shifting astral form, but maintained a steady gaze which seemed impartial or unattached, yet at the same time was willing to be present and perhaps even curious. I strive to not want anything from the Queen Devi and she seems to not want from me. My meditation was filled with the thoughts about how any strange or alien sentience elicits fear in some people, especially those who are irrational and superstitious. The Queen Devi is stable in her vast power and there is nothing a mortal can do to her. I feel gratitude that she would spend any attention on a mere mortal human who seeks an audience with her. Her presence is all knowing and pure being in the light that is enlightening, humbling, and healing.
    At one point I saw an alligator and recalled seeing one in my dream last night. Though my wife mentioned one last evening, somehow the image was empowered to return out of many things mentioned. Alligators are ancient beasts with a core need for water and yet who like the fiery hot sun as well. Perhaps the Queen Devi is indicating a boundary area of astral space where we are encountering each other. Traditionally Fire and Water balance each other and when balanced represent good health: physically, mentally, and emotionally.
    I also saw the spatial form of blue with a pulsating red dot and then it was transformed into green with a pulsating yellow dot. This was interspersed with thoughts arising about engaging a presence. Then the four colors seemed to wrap up in a ball and form a Turquoise Pearl which vibrated in an expanding and contracting mode and yet expanding was dominant and it grew large and had a smooth wet luster. It was extremely aesthetically pleasing and seemed to express an elegant beauty. This brought to my mind the two archetypal Blue Princesses, the Sweet Princess Devi and the Fierce Princess Devi. They

are both so much more humanoid and so beautiful and attractive. They serve the Queen Devi and she uses them as her intermediaries. The Turquoise Pearl symbolized their beauty as a precious treasure which can rejuvenate life force.

I also saw the Mandorla (almond shape) also known as vesica piscis (referring to a lens shape) made by two circles of the same size interacting. The interior of the circles was red, while the intersection was blue. The intersection lens then took on a primary importance as the circles mutated to be the space which held the lens. This was like a body holding the inner more refined soul of Consciousness. It invited the sense of a portal without any thoughts arising in my mind and indicated that each person is a portal and the inner gateway can be opened to travel upon. The image was indeed organic and spoke of the sacred nature of the union of two beings and the pulsation of life force that is shared. **In any encounter, interaction, or communication we exchange energy and our personal sense of being includes something of the other.** If we dialog with clarity about something of importance, we grow intellectually, learning and teaching.

To be aware of the Queen Devi's presence is very humbling and yet empowering. One must be ready to be in Her sentient presence with no secrets to hide, totally naked on all levels and in the most subtle expressions which one radiates. The Queen Devi is transparent and her presence is like the presence of the natural mystery of the Cosmos. At the same time She is a divine mirror revealing the essence rather than the superficial.

Session 0054:

Aim Klim Sauh: In-Breath Aim, Out-Breath Mmm (a subtle continuance), In-Breath Kleem, Out-Breath Mmm (a subtle continuance), In-Breath Sow, Out-Breath aHhhh (a subtle continuance),

    I choose this seed Sundari mantra. My first impression was a fish in a clear plastic bag, as if one just purchased it and will float the bag in one's fish tank until the temperatures match, then add the fish to the tank. I am not formally in any meditation group, religion, or cult and yet there is acceptance by all true meditation practitioners of anyone using a method that works and adding awareness in the collective field of humanity and the Earth. Sometimes there is a desire to indoctrinate or sell classes, and often if I do not join a group and they stop inviting me or exclude content from me, indicating that they are stuck in the failing paradigm of exclusivity. I am not saying that a humble donation to support facilitators is unacceptable, but to learn to meditate just requires doing it and that does not cost anything; so, just do it.

    I then briefly sensed the two eyes of a Queen Devi and within the blackness there were multicolored spirals. The face morphed until I saw faces of the a Princess Blue Devi. Her face changed and eventually was not similar to a human, but was still feminine. There was a conveyed sense as if asking if I still liked her appearance and I assured her it was attractive and I was not going to judge her for her physical form. She then became a beautiful turquoise color and I saw her embracing a white human male (pure white like paper). I think the image was shown to teach how she contrasted various appearances and yet she got no emotional response from me in meditation. Her face then darkened and became blue-black with her slightly strange featured qualities and then she faded.

    I then sensed space opening to the larger astral realm and sensed a lot of activity there. There were all kinds of dreamers there from around the galaxy, engaged in their various quests, mostly unaware of each other. **In meditation one is in a mode where contact with higher beings is possible and yet very difficult.** There is a vastness of much more space and the space is much more fluid. **One needs strong discernment when engaging any other being, just like choosing which humans to spend time and energy with.** Intent to only meet beneficent beings is useful, but does not assure that every being one will encounter will have spiritual intent. One's energy must remain clear and not be able to be enticed by adventure.

Sometimes Shim, Shrim, or Hum was be added to my mental chanting with my breath. This is all fine when it happens spontaneously and when one is deep, one only somewhat notices the shift. These added their character and helped me balance in my heart. I did not feel inclined to formally send energy to anyone or pick up any individuals energy, but rather sensed the larger group of humans all over the Earth meditating. **As more people on the planet meditate, everyone goes deeper and has more energetic experiences.** In meditation one feels connection to all of humanity, but special connection to others who are meditating. We all benefit from each other's dedication to increasing our awareness through meditation. In this sense meditating is a service to all of humanity.

Session 0055:

Lakshmi: Out-Breath Lah, in the pause after the exhale and before the inhale an almost silent 'K', In-Breath Shmee.

 The question of what is real wealth arises with Lakshmi. Good health is a great wealth, without which other aspects of life are diminished. The requirements for the body must be present to maintain good health, but excess is actually contrary to good health. Then there is affection, a loving partner is a richness that is superb and a family group which is spiritual in orientation is a rich asset. All the things one has will be sacrificed as one dies, therefore what is lasting wealth? This is an open question deserving deep contemplation.

 As I meditated deeper I came to realize that the 'k' needed to be subtle and connected to the pause after the exhale, grounded at the root and connecting one to the Earth. The Earth is a vast treasure and provides all that we have and we all will return all form to the Earth. I then saw a headband with a jewel in the center like a diamond shape descending to cover the third eye. A clear mind and astute discrimination is a very fine treasure, a jewel which provides one the means to choose one's path in a way that fulfills the deeper needs of one's life. Then I saw a dancing goddess as a body moving. It was a golden yellow cluster of luminous strings, a glowing form which exemplified fluid movement. **The dance of life is a treasure, a precious gift from the Cosmos.**

 Then the mantra became faint as it became more steady and natural. This is a deeper level where the will to focus on the mantra fades and the mantra has its own momentum, it is said that it comes alive. It is just like breathing which we do not need to maintain, since the Cosmos is breathing us. The phone rang with an errand required, I was interrupted and so I went and did the task. On returning to meditation I added Kali:

Lakshmi Kali: Out-Breath Lah, in the pause an almost silent 'K', In-Breath Shmee., Out-Breath Kah, In-Breath Lee.

 The left field of astral vision and right field of astral vision were separated by a line with the red on the left and yellow on the right. I had the impression of the division of the living from the dead. This was followed by being in a room where a movie or play was about to begin. It was very crowded, but a few chairs were added and they were up front and center. A new family was seated in them. Already seated was a boy child hanging out of his seat, not focused on the proceedings for the coming play. In that Kali, Goddess of Time, added the question about what remains after death and the message is that we react to the contents of the play. **All our choices and the feelings we radiate are the treasure or garbage we carry with us.**

   I then saw an Egyptian eye and as the eye faded I felt the fading of ancient Egypt. Then I saw a reptile's eye and sensed the fading of countless species of dinosaurs. I then saw a flying saucer radiating a beam of light down, which became a showering of drops of souls. This was followed by a tall bird's eye and a sea mammal's eye, both now extinct. In reference to the flying saucer I will admit that I have read a lot of literature in reference to the extra-terrestrial presence on the Earth and think it is a strong probability that they monitor and record Earth's evolution and possibly interject influences; however I cannot do more than report the flow of the meditation. Whether it is an indication of something real or a reflection of my thinking, I do not know, but I can state definitely that the course of the meditation followed the nature of the mantra in theme and content.

   Then I found myself chanting Shakti which is very similar to Lakshmi and after several variations was chanting Kali Shakti Lakshmi Hum: Time, Energy, Wealth, the Spiritual Heart. I then saw a tiger, a powerful predator and often goddess Durga is symbolized in graphics as riding a tiger and represents protection. **While a fierce image, the protection of the Cosmos for its ongoing and transforming creation is a natural fact: the Cosmos evolves more conscious beings by design.** Then before me flashed powerful people who are now history and who are now forgotten. Nothing survives Kali, the ongoing rush of time: all that is gets recycled into something new. Lasting wealth maybe very ambiguous to conceive of but somehow I sense that all that can be attained is a more conscious state in the now and an accumulation of memories of a life well lived which make the present a rich journey.

Session 0056:

Kali Ma Akasha Hum: Out-Breath Kah, In-Breath Lee, Out-Breath Mah, In-Breath Ah, Out-Breath Kash, In-Breath Ah, Out-Breath Hum, In-Breath Silence.

    Sometimes I wake at 3 AM and lay in bed doing mantra. These meditations are not documented here because the mantra changes and I drift into and out of deep sleep without anything mental, only work in the luminous which is beyond astral or void. Last night I composed this mantra for Kali, Goddess of Time, and Akasha, infinite Space, and Hum for heart and the way it works it actually contains Ahum, I Am, my own being spending time in space. I had a vision that was relevant which was of a navel which had an energetic whirlpool descending into the depths of my being and from the center of the vortex was a counter directional spiral being emitted with power. The inward spiral may represent 'gut-feelings' in which the outward spiral represents the personal power of the force of curved space connecting to the Earth and Cosmos.
    In this meditation I perceived an energy separating the positive curvature from the negative curvature and thus creating the tension or torque between the two geometries. The material aspect of the Cosmos is based upon this torque. The red is below and vibrates slow and the blue above and vibrates fast and so there is a spectrum of separation in the field of astral light. I then saw two red dots and saw that beyond the spectrum, in each vibration there is a duality as time unwinds the energy.
    This was followed by seeing the womb as the space where the soul enters and accumulates space by curving it around its axis. The sperm splits the egg and it starts a chain reaction of dividing. I then felt very clearly the tactile sensation of reaching out with my hand and touching denim cloth, the texture of the weave, and this sensation is perhaps how the illusion of boundary is conceived/woven. I was meditating and not touching anything, this was astral sensation that felt totally real. **In the body, the inner space matches the outer space of the entire Cosmos.** This is the profound potency of every beings inner space, which reflects a unique perspective of the Cosmos. Over the course of the meditation I saw a vision of an axe splitting a log (as a sperm splits an egg) and also of opening the seal of a baggie to have space within it and be able to be filled. Since numerous visions returned on this theme, the manner in which space is opened, exemplified that two parts are created from one

and then there is expansion which creates room for form in the space between.

I saw an upward pointing triangle formed of points of light, first one at the peak, then two below that, then more and more; such that, as the triangle ascended there were increasing numbers of points of light. This is the nature of the creation of a body depicted in two dimensions, as the body forms and grows. **I was also shown that when One splits into two (time and space), each of the two parts contains the pattern of the One.** The pattern exists in both realms. Perhaps time has patterns which are similar, though inverted, relative to the forms of space and thereby there is the momentum of the tension as time transforms all spatial form.

Then I was presented with death and the dissolution of form. I considered in meditation that there are two realms, the realm of the living and the realm of the dead and that the celestial realm is the unifying energy which holds them both within its patterns. It seemed as if the splitting of the egg separated the I Am of my total being and set a boundary between these two realms. One's celestial nature binds them and the transformation of space which was created in separation of the personal I Am from the cosmic I Am which continuously exists as one bounces in a vibratory manner from life in this realm to life among the dead. A higher dimensional connective force (I Am) exists such that space and time are dependent upon each other and cannot exist without each other; space vibrates - time cycles.

These were the impressions of this meditation which then presented me with a profound question: "Why did you choose the parents you chose to bring you into this life?" Not hearing a voice, but rather the question downloaded complete in my mind and my response was that this will be a very hard question to answer. Coming out of meditation I must seriously ponder that question: somehow when the male energy opened the space-time within the female energy and opened the door between the two sides, their union gave me a birth into the experience of space-time existing. The third element is energy, the momentum and will of the life tree to expand and evolve. **This trinity should be addressed as Time-Energy-Space rather than the duality of space-time.** Within every person there is a deep longing to grow, to seek to be more, and understand something of the infinite mystery of the Cosmos within which we live. This is a profound energy, our spirit, which we may harness and express as the spiral of our lives which we emit with every intent and choice we make.

Session 0057:

Aum Kali Kala Sauh: Out-Breath Ah, In-Breath Mmm (a subtle continuance), Out-Breath Kah, In-Breath Lee, Out-Breath Kah, In-Breath Lah, Out-Breath Sa, In-Breath Uh.

 The choice of mantra is somewhat spontaneous and I do not know what motivates a choice, I just listen to my predilection in the now. I had many visions from around the world as well as the tendency to go deep and find my head bobbing down in relaxation. **Our interconnections exist beyond time-space-energy within the higher dimensionality I refer to as the celestial realm.** Humanity is an organ of the Earth in the same way the brain is an organ of the body. Organs must be balanced within the totality of the higher body they fit within.
 The first sensation was of 'Welcome to Hawaii' and I sensed a number of people were gathered there (I have never been there). This was followed by a scene around a spring fed pool of clear water. There were people with flowers and a sense of celebration. Then I heard a voice saying [a first name] is climbing up the stairs. Perhaps this was a celebration of life ceremony.
 Then I sensed 'I don't want to watch Olympic games anymore'; and the impression that I got was that all competition sports training for war and are slowly losing the attention of people. The new focus which can hold people's attention is nature based cooperation of life doing service and the attaining of great benefit for humanity. I had a brief flash of sitting outside, in front of a restaurant, and discussing deep philosophy or science with some people and then I was in a hanger. There was a cutting edge hypersonic space plane there. I realize that the next frontier for humanity is space exploration. Humans are explorers by nature and that could be the ultimate attractive viewing: the reality of men and women exploring the solar system and setting up bases and colonies. The video feeds would need to be intimate and reveal the tremendous psychological challenges of traversing the void and living upon deadly planets, but also the richly rewarding new discoveries and amazing sights.
 I then saw an executive man, one who had enough power and wealth to be dressed somewhat casual and yet still exude his position of authority. I gave him a little push on his shoulder and he reacted and looked at me in shock, because I was not really there. I slipped a key card set into his pocket and then I manifest my face and stared at him. I do not know who he was, but perhaps now he understands that the

humans with the keys are not the personality types these organizations are seeking and therefore they are missing the greatest thinkers. The people have an inner commitment to freedom and can provide the tools for ethical technology to take humanity to the stars.

Humanity is at a delicate crossroad and change in inevitable. Some of my interpretation here was only sensed in the meditation. Aum is the essence of Consciousness, as individuals and as the collective of humanity and the Earth. Kali is the Goddess of time and Kala is time itself, the dividing and measuring cycles within cycles within which the fluctuating changes flow. Sauh is the passion, the most intimate curiosity and the need to expand beyond that which is limiting, the quest for freedom. Kali and Kala are like lovers, balancing each other in their union to be more than their sum. Therefore this mantra seemed to drive towards big changes for humanity. None of the imagery was expected or anticipated. Some of the interpretation is based on analyzing feelings and general intuitive impressions that were received in the meditation.

Session 0058:

Bhairavi Bhairava: Out-Breath Bhai (Bh has a popping explosive nature followed by a sound like the word eye; altogether more coming from the heart/chest center more than the word bye), In-Breath Rahvee, Out-Breath Bhai, In-Breath Rahvah

Interestingly the first impression I got was that of Bhairavi being like water, continuous and steady and Bhairava being like the wind, expressing itself as powerful gusts which impact and fade in repetitive phases. This was followed by Bhairavi as the whole Cosmos holding within Bhairava, the Consciousness which illuminates. This was followed by two chevron shapes, like boomerangs, which were overlapped in the center. This is an alternative to two isosceles triangles overlapping and presents each force as having an orientation toward and into each other. Post meditation I can consider both space and time as the chevrons and their intersection is the Cosmos total energy/mass ($e/c + mc$). **Together Bhairavi and Bhairava create the play of transforming form where they touch and overlap.**

Then as the other more open dimension became available to my awareness, I perceived the face of an old shamanic man with an intense gaze, as if wondering who I am, perhaps even waiting for me or whomever might find their way to the other realm. Then I perceived a left hand upon a sphere and the sphere represented Earth or was the Earth. I also perceived the classic image of women which we see in the ancient Goddess statues and this was followed by a squatting woman's form which implies giving birth. I felt the energy of protectors, warriors dedicated to the life of the Earth. **There is a rebirthing of what humanity is, in progress at this time.**

Mixed with this succession of images I saw an old metal Buddha incense burner which I had from before I was a teenager, but which I used to burn incense in as a teenager. I am not sure where I got it from. The question of 'What did they do to me as a child?' arose, without any clarity of who the 'they' referred to or which specific traumatic experience this might refer to. There was an intensity of impact upon me as a youth from a young age which caused me to question everything. I know many young people do not feel as if they fit in, but I could not understand our culture to the point of not trying to fit in because too many things made no sense. Therefore I was an intense spiritual seeker and started mantra meditation in my early teens (more than fifty years ago).

I then saw patterns in light blue lines as on a white plate. These were tree like in their fractal branching and kept shifting and transforming in patterns which had symmetry. At one point they became three dimensional and were incomprehensible, thus I cannot recall them clearly, for they were beyond what ordinary vision beholds. This again made me feel the open space. The feeling was as if I was sliding or floating and I had a vertigo sensation associated with the sense of motion. This had occurred several times in the meditation and was now stronger, as if my axis of perception was going to fall out of the Cosmos and into this open dimension. There was no fear, but rather an overall sensation of bliss. Indeed I felt as if I was pulsations within a superb energy, a subtle emotional radiance which was pleasurable and transcended the limitations of my bodily form, of which I was only vaguely aware.

Session 0059:

Shiva Shakti Akasha: In-Breath She, Out-Breath Vah, In-Breath Shak, Out-Breath Tee, In-Breath Ah, Out-Breath Kah, In-Breath Shah, Out-Breath Ha (a subtle continuance; occasionally Hum / Hoom).

Right away space opened and this is perhaps in relation to Akasha, meaning space or ether, which also contains all the vibrations of the past. Then from the right lower corner of my astral vision a round faced blue male image appeared with a red mark upon his forehead. He radiated gladness and satisfaction. I took it as a positive sign for this mantra meditation. I then perceived things roiling below the surface, intense and powerful energies not yet present in my conscious awareness, but very active.

The second and sixth centers were activated and I saw numerous astral images suggesting how space, time, and energy were related. The first was a circle with red to the left and blue to the right. Two chevron shapes had their points overlapping the circle and thereby creating three sections. The blue seemed to be higher in frequency than the red and so while both sides had both colors as small energy vibrations the blue seemed to move more. Then I saw a circle of mostly blue with a center line of mostly red dividing it vertically into two halves, but each half also had a mostly red dot. Again the energy was scintillating with the colors.

The next image was of a strainer and the more fine liquid stuff moving through it faster and the denser, more gelatinous liquid moving slowly and being the end of the contents moving through the strainer. This was followed by a glass of liquid of different densities settling into layers. The next image was of a Shiva lingam stone in blue and a red sunset sky behind it. I did not see any base or lower area, which is where the roiling vibrations were sensed. This mutated until the blue lingam was a smooth dome and could only be seen from the right as bright blue light and the left was obscured in the bottom flat end of the bright blue column and the rounded top was a doorway. It was sensed as a door, but was obscured and was part of the left aspect which was hidden.

Then I saw a loaf of bread rising with yeast bubbles within it. This was followed by the sense of several colloidal images where very fine bubbles of one substance were dispersed within either a liquid or a solid. These gave way to the sensation that these bubbles were eating the substrate of the matrix. Following this I sensed a complex concept beyond visuals of the two components (the red and blue) having been thoroughly mixed in a unified whole being and then being separated and in the coming apart there was diversity of form.

These last three paragraphs contain a very complex and dynamic symbolic representation of Time, Space, and the resultant Energy in the center. The Trisula (Trident) or Trinity of all that is. The cosmic principles of (red) Space falling through (blue) Time causes a vibration within every point of space-time at the most subtle Plank scale and from the vibration there arises Energy (and mass is just farther separated or collapsed Energy: mc = e/c). **Space is a positive curvature falling through Time, which can be considered the opposite or negative curvature, and like a violin bow on a string, there is generated a vibrational hum, a radiant sound, the ultimate Word, from which the entire Cosmos is emitted.** Energy is high vibration interaction of contact where Space falls through Time. Matter is like tiny bubbles of vibrational standing waves in the matrix of Time.

I perceived a yellow sphere and it reminded me of our radiant sun, but I knew there was more significance. I felt a very deep and profound passion, sensual and yet not erotic, very deeply human, a longing and a drive. I saw the yellow sphere's surface bubbling up from below and layers of bubbles pushed up as new bubbled were emitted. The upper layer would sometimes pop and break down as the newer layers moved up in response to yet more new layers. At this point I also sensed a very fierce and powerful protection for the way of life. A warrior spirit which would prevail against the forces of chaos and continue to create the manifestation of ever more aware life and to support and sustain life's elements until it was time to reabsorb them. I perceived a very old manuscript and knew it contained wonderful esoteric wisdom, but it was yellowing and crumbling away.

Nothing lasts in Energy or Matter, but in the patterns of space, ether, or primary geometry etched by Time there are deep feelings being embedded. When we meditate we generate a radiance of the nectar of bliss. To conclude the meditation and ground back in the body I was presented with the technique of sending some of that higher vibrational humming radiance of bliss to a loved one. It will be healing for them and return me to the human life. Life is a personal expression of that divine dance of Time, perceived as Consciousness, embracing Space, perceived as the Sentient Mystery, moving as the Cosmos of energy-matter ever-changing form. **Using our will to focus our intent and direct the higher vibration in compassionate love is the most supreme work which humanity may engage in and meditation is the** key to intensifying the vibration and potentiating it to raise the collective whole of humanity.

Session 0060:

Klim Hrim Srim Im: In-Breath Kleem, Out-Breath Mmm (a subtle continuance),In-Breath Hreem, Out-Breath Mmm (a subtle continuance), In-Breath Shreem, Out-Breath Mmm (a subtle continuance), In-Breath Eem, Out-Breath Mmm (a subtle continuance).

The universe I live in, my reality, world view, or paradigm is a copy of what is there, with less detail and some errors added. As I was contemplating this while existing in open astral space, a gloved hand put into my hand something which seemed like the pull top of a can. Since I was in the dream state, but fully conscious, I felt this sensation. This is profound because up until now the dreaming energy has been mostly visual with some thought sounds interjected. Interpreting this I would say that some garbage perceptual information is handed to me by the human form, garbage based upon a mental conception of the Cosmos as opposed to a direct perception. I need to consciously find ways to discard the perceptual errors which will result in my gaining a better knowing of the Mystery within which I am a conscious perceiver and active participant.

Then I saw a sacred woman in blue robes, which is a Christian iconic image. The image radiated femininity and was supremely attractive in an awe inspiring manner. It quickly faded which left me with the desire of a hug, a conversation, or even another instant of her awareness. The message was to purify the mind and see the Goddess in a holistic manner, which is not in a physical manner. This does not refer to sexual energy because that was not the feeling existing, but rather that any person is more of a complex personality than the mind can grasp. We cannot even grasp our personal selves. In modern times we humans tend to live in our heads. While the person is not the constructed personality with its conditioned elements of self-identity or ego, yet that ego is what interacts emotionally in our daily world. A higher being would be living from the vantage point of pure Consciousness, and would perceive their personality as constructed ego engaging in the dance of life, the play of form within the Mystery of the manifest Cosmos, rather than their true self.

My wife and I live on a small hobby farm and the animals became present in my awareness. We have a mean old goose which acts as a watchdog and somewhat protection for our small flock of ducks. The message came through that the goose's fear based reality does not allow a good reading of reality. This is perspective since from a higher

Goddess's point of view my human reading of reality would not be good either. I lock the ducks in a shed at night, since they are easy prey and in the meditation I was showing someone how I do this. The ducks generally listen to me telling them to go home if it is twilight or has gotten dark. I can act as a guardian for their lives even if I cannot be a friend or have much interaction. **I sense that there are presences which act as guardians for us and our world.** I feel that I must consider with careful evaluation all methodologies for gaining increased awareness as potentially valid processes to pursue getting over conditioned illusions in life.

 We also have a few rare breed Soay sheep. I sold most of them and have three weathers (fixed males) left since I am getting old and minimizing chores. They have a natural tendency to fear, even though in some ways they want to be friends. Their nature does not include touching and so they stay six feet away from me. I seek to work with them and overcome their natural tendency. I feed them hay and I feel safe being around them, even though they sometimes ram each other: horns to horns. Does the Goddess have offerings for me and do I need to make her feel safe for her to enter more powerfully in my astral perception? I am meditating to learn. Even if it is all my 'subconscious' dreaming these things, what do I need to do to invite deeper interaction and more rich experience with the subtle aspects of the sentient Cosmos?

 I then had the sense of more people in our society seeking to alleviate their fears by buying guns. Their fear having grown to pathological levels, they no longer would accept any extra-terrestrial presence, which is now confirmed to be present on Earth. The number of people living by scamming others and the institutionalization of corporate deception, which is deeply affecting people's lives, leads to a mental state where the perceived universe is always assumed to be hostile. Fear of the other, of any unfamiliar presence, does not lead to expanding networks of cooperative functionality. I then saw a man looking under the hood of his broken down pick-up truck. This symbol seems appropriate for the end result of fear based realty which goes far beyond cautious discrimination and results in breakdown.

 I play a vertical bamboo Shakuhachi flute. Sometimes I play for the sheep, who react to my initial presence, but then graze peacefully with me in the field with them. Some Shakuhachi flutes can play higher notes in the third octave easier than others and some people are more skilled at attaining the higher notes: practice is the key. Meditation is like this in that some people are more capable of stilling their mind and sinking into the astral dream state while remaining lucid and taking a trip in the subtle inner spaces which open up. There is an element of practice and no beginner should expect dramatic results, but with years of practice one comes to very rich and deep exploration. **The images which become present as mantra thought sounds are encountered are filled with the essence of a subtle layer of meaning which are the essence of sacred vibrations.** The impressions of meanings being conveyed in the images and sounds as I describing the experience I am clarifying by adding commentary based upon that set of intuitive feelings.

I then sensed my bodily form as a set of boundaries that was pulsating with my breath. I was breathing in blue light and exhaling red luminous energy. **My body was lit up and the Cosmos was breathing me! I pondered how a cosmic fluctuation could be breathing me, when other animals breathe at different rates and was intuitively informed that the different bodily forms catch the cosmic pulsation differently.** Then I held my breath, but of course I had to release it, therefore the nature of the cosmic pulsation, the rising and falling wave within which I exist, provides a momentum to live and breathe. **The vibrations of the geometry of space itself potentiates breath!**

Then I was translocated and found myself within a room with large windows covered by light curtains which had symbols on them. There was a keyboard in the room and a desk. It was an office and workspace, but a distraction in daily life brought me out of meditation. The room was significant because it was more like lucid dreaming, where my pulsating dream body had found a dream space and my human form was functional. It seems every meditation leaves one with enticements by showing there is so much more to encounter in future meditation adventures.

Session 0061:

Sauh: In-Breath Sow, Out-Breath Ahh (Very subtle fading H sound).

    I realize right away that the mantric sound of breath (Sah inhale and Ahh exhale) are combined at the pause between in-breath and out-breath with the 'au' vowel sound: making it related to SoHam or HamSa (Ham is like English Hum), the natural sound of breath.
    The first astral image is of a lens shaped black portal opening in the floor, surrounded by layers of color. Then the illumination of my bodily form within the astral realm. There is a sense of energy flow, into and out of the bodily boundary. As breath and energy cycle a hum of radiance flows out and around my bodily form. Unlike some misconceptions, the astral realm is a very sensual place. It is not grounded like the physical and so has a subtler level of interaction and yet also a freer nature with more possibilities. I then saw the two overlapped chevron shapes from left and right with their points overlapping and also forming the lens shape in their intersection.
    I briefly saw a pair of pink farm books, a woman walking the path in nature is implied. There is a sexual nature to this mantra and to all of creation. This energy reflects the sense of duality coming together for unity. In the astral realm sexuality is not as limited as it is in the physical realm, but takes on higher elements. I sensed the Wild Blue Devi appearing in several fierce forms, as if teasing me with strange faces to see if I would want the being behind those faces. This brought up the thought of the mantra Kali.
    At this point something very profound occurred. While the mantra with my breath was clearly the thought vibration Sauh, as if I was saying it clearly in my thoughts, overlapped in subtle form was Kali, as a layer of thought energy more subtle that actual thoughts. While doing the inhale and exhale with Sauh I was simultaneously doing Kali, but not as thoughts pronounced, rather as thoughts intended and subtly being thought. **This brings awareness to how one can be chanting a mantra in one's thoughts while simultaneously the ideas behind thoughts can pass through the mind silently.** The most vocal or loudest thought was Sauh, while the thought idea was Kali. This implies that even in ordinary waking state one may be thinking a set of words and an idea may arise as an overlay; both stories occurring simultaneously. Kali had some movement to take over the top mantra position, but I maintained my intended mantra and Kali accepted the

more subtle sphere of pure idea energy. Both mantras were simultaneous, but operating on different frequencies of my mind.

Session 0062:

Shakti Shiva: In-Breath Shock, Out-Breath Tee, In-Breath Shee, Out-Breath Vah

Shakti is the Cosmos, its order and the continuing sentient creative expression thereof. Shiva is Consciousness, the sentience of every living thing. I started by seeing a blue woman to the right and a red field to the left. Hearing the word Ishvara, the personality of the divine transcendental, I understood that this represented the fact that the Cosmos has a unique relationship to every person. We have mental impressions which obscure the true nature of the vast informational flux of the Cosmos, but when we recognize a synchronicity we know that it is intimately wise about our personal life. Therefore the personification of the Cosmic sentience is a natural human tendency, but it is much more complex than that.

Then I saw a vertical sign which was lit up with a single strand of writing from top to bottom. As I looked closer this was shakuhachi flute music, which I read and play daily, but I was unable to read the specifics of the tune. There is a data stream flowing through my Consciousness like notes of music flowing by a listener: the song is interpreted through remembering what has past and riding the present with a trailing memory of notes lingering. Speech has the same characteristic, sound is present, but the string of words in the memory convey a meaning. **Without memory, there is no song or meaning, only sound.**

Then there was a vision of a hat with silverware on it. Shakti has a sense of humor and is informing my Consciousness that I am feeding my mind all kinds of things, I need to remember that these impressions stick and my sense of self is influenced. The hat morphed into an image of Saturn and its rings, which is a symbol of Karma, not a simplistic eye for eye, but one must live with themselves, with all their acts and thoughts, and the impressions which they have embraced and radiated. I then saw a blue God like male figure holding a wicker basket by the handle. This would represent me and all living beings being carried down the river of time with stuff pouring in and running out through the holes. We hold onto things briefly and then, like our mortal bodies, they return to the Cosmos.

A red masculine face then appeared. I was informed to balance within the torrents of time cascading through me. The blue representing Shakti (the perceived Cosmos) and red representing Shiva (life's perceiving Consciousness) is reversed in the real nature, Shakti precedes Shiva, for the Cosmos as a mysterious unknown, a dark void filled with everything, and awakens Consciousness within it, to illuminate aspects of itself, sustaining that Consciousness for being's many lifespans, and then reabsorbing all that is created and the Consciousness back into herself as aspects of her supreme Consciousness.

A yellow field of Shiva light of Consciousness in my dreaming mind's eye was then inhabited by a green Shakti Goddess image dancing. The red and blue symbology of my inner being elucidated upon by my meditation astral images as external (yellow) time - Consciousness and (green) space - Cosmos. Then there was a glass door from inside a house to outside and rather than looking out I saw the door being removed and the outer scent of the air and the sounds of nature flowing in. **A human form is very permeable and the mind constructs boundaries which are resistance to direct perception, to Consciousness truly dancing with the Cosmos.**

At this point I realized the need to honor the Trisula, the Trinity, space and time touching and united in central point of energy (which incorporates mass): the trinity as all that is rather than duality as a basis of understanding the Unity. It is the interaction of positive space falling through negative time, Shiva Consciousness penetrating the mystery of Shakti, which gives rise to the unified totality of all of creation. I therefore added the mantra Aum reversed (Breathe in Ahhh and breathe out Mmmm fading into silence) as a third aspect of Shakti being united with Shiva, as Yin and Yang are united in the circle of the Way, Tao.

I then saw a burlap sack of yellow corn with green lettering: the inside contents of what is held in Consciousness was visible from the outside, but the green lettering, the detailed information is a mental overlay, a description which lacks the detail of the direct sensory perception of the course weave of the fabric and the color and essence of the inner grain. Then I saw blue writing upon red, inner space being harder to read as the colors play games together, the perceiver and the perceived are not distinct, though the mind functions with such duality, the overlap of pure perceiving is the third aspect and closer to unity. I saw a red dot, a point of space, a Plank unit, within a halo of blue field of Consciousness. **Space holds energy-mass falling through time: our bodies fall into the future driven by an insatiable impulse and so our bodies are not nouns, they are ever changing verbs.**

This was followed by a curtain with vertical red and blue stripes and with a slight translucence, behind which the Goddess Shakti was dancing naked and she was looking at me. I sense some sentient information which is invisible and beyond description and is the ordering of the dance of the totality and yet which is personally and intimately relating to every being in their life journey. I received a message that it was wonderful when a group of humans formed a circle. This represented the merging of our Consciousness toward a unified goal of comprehending the totality of the Cosmos of energy, not just mentally, but experientially. It implies humans meditating all over the planet and the Consciousness of each person meditating being amplified exponentially.

Then I saw the Queen Devi and she indicated the truth was beyond form and therefore any symbols used, any poetic words rendered, can only hint at the truth. Then a saw a book laying open with yellow pages and green writing. This is a repeat of the bag of corn symbology and so significant. A flash of a human Yogini (a female Yoga master) with eyes that were yellow with green lines radiating from their centers. Then the statement, 'I ordered them for you.'. Some of this relates to a dream I had last night, where I met a woman who was a Yogini and at the end she looked in my eyes, but in the dream after looking into her eyes, then I only saw one eye as a circle mandala with soft green lines in the iris filling my whole vision. All I can say is that we see spatial form in continual change and intuit time, but time itself seems formless, as does Consciousness.

Then I saw a stairway in a building which descended into darkness far below. There were no landings as if it switched back and forth, but rather it seemed like a continual tunnel of stairs descending into the darkness. This was followed by an aerial view as if flying low over fields. forest, and a river. There appeared to be country roads, but no town, nor did I see houses in my short viewing of perhaps a mile or so. Our Consciousness shines down into the darkness and the farther we seek to illuminate, the darker it gets, just as in my aerial view looking down which lacked detail and was also moving by at a quick pace, such that I could only see so much detail, but many specifics were not perceivable. There is vast multidimensional aspects of the Cosmos flowing around us unseen. There is much greater darkness, the vastness of what our Consciousness cannot illuminate, than there is what is experienced in our perceived time tunnel of life.

The final vision is described as most flute players have their instruments wrapped up in a colored cloth bag as a blanket of protection. As a shakuhachi flute player this is a global message about music and about life. Most musicians dress up their music and use hooks to catch people's attention as they seek popularity. A detailed blanket is not warmer or more beautiful than one with minimalistic designs. The shakuhachi flute repertoire includes ancient Zen music and we who incorporate this musical tradition seek pure tone and honest expression in our music. **Authenticity has more elegance than glamorous flashiness. The ever flowing design of the touch of Shakti, the sentience of the Cosmos, is elegant.** The darkness hides mysteries and entices Consciousness to intensify with a longing for the secret ecstasy which is dancing behind the curtain of energetic form: to embrace the essence that twinkles in the eyes, and to know Cosmic Union.

Session 0063:

Aum Shakti Shiva: out-Breath A(uw)hh, In-Breath (u)Mmm (a subtle continuance), Out-Breath Shock, In-Breath Tee, Out-Breath She, In-Breath Vah.

First a door opening to descending stairs, going deeper within myself I briefly sensed a blue male to my left giving me a brief hand over my shoulder. Since I had no body at the time, it was somewhat of a symbol in astral space, rather than a tactile impression. Then the sky was the rich blue of time and below was the deep red of space. In the sky a starburst of blue flashed. Following this I sensed my physical body as if energy was coursing through it and it felt very light, as if it could begin to float, but I stayed grounded.

Then a sentence came through about a man who has been very sick and the message was 'If I see them, there is something I am supposed to do.' Following which I perceived a succession of lifetimes with some pauses between. This is a clarification that we carry trauma from the deep past, as well as joyous memories, and also that we have a unique nature which transcends cultural conditioning and the effects of what we experience in each life. I then saw green bananas turning yellow and then getting spots, I can understand this as the progression of time on a biological body, we all age and die. What remains is the impressions we focus on. Memories, even deep past life memories, can arise in the present, but it is our choice to reinforce them or let them fade away.

I then saw a blue woman dancing in space, it was her very feminine form moving with grace. This is Shakti enticing Shiva, the Cosmos teasing Consciousness into a heightened state. As conscious beings we become the seekers, the searchers, the ones looking for the ultimate wisdom and for peace. Shakti proceeds Shiva and is forever wise and powerful and Shiva is always one step behind.

Then I saw the blue man go through the gate, offering me to follow and saying, 'You pay for the rest of it yourself.' One can read all the scriptures and do all the practices, but one must truly experience transcendental wisdom to know it. Mentally understanding and knowing all the practices is the offer to go through the gate, but to actually go through the gate, one must face the sacred Mystery completely revealed, having offered one's life in payment for freedom. I then saw a group of diverse children watching the play at the gate with the curious intensity of innocent wonder. There is nothing which remains hidden in any of one's activities or thoughts when one gets to the gate.

Finally I saw a Blue Devi, not the supreme, but a semi-immortal being of very high nature, extremely powerful, indicating that she can only offer me so much because there are those with base power whom she cannot overrule. There is a war in the heavens, a power struggle which seems so immature, yet seems to be the nature of the forces playing games with humanity. The message is that each one of us must assume our personal power and collectively claim our right to being a sovereign being in order for humanity to become a sovereign species.

Following this I saw patterns like the winged heart and the convex lens shape of the sacred portal. These were continually transforming with other geometric shapes faster than my mind could get a handle on them to remember them. At this point I realized my breath was very faint, slow and distant, while my body was vague and space was open inside and out, lacking clear distinction. I was floating in bliss and knew that bliss is the ultimate inheritance, but it is an intensely conscious ecstatic bliss, rather than a dull sleepy state.

Session 0064:

Aum Bhagavati Devi: Out-Breath Aum, In-Breath Mmm (a subtle continuance), Out-Breath Bhah, In-Breath Gah, Out-Breath Vah, In-Breath Tee, Out-Breath Deh, In-Breath Vee,

There is a technique in Chi Gong where one holds their hands in front of their abdomen with palms facing and separating them while breathing in and bringing them close together while breathing out, gradually moving them farther apart while the energy between them accumulates. This forms a Chi Ball, or an accumulation of pranic life force, in the space between the hands which can then be placed in the body for energy or healing. **I saw in this meditation that as we breath, our body is doing the same process of accumulating Chi, Prana, higher dimensional life force, or the water of life (pick your favorite label).** This is a profound realization about how breathing with intention is a primary means of healing and also why meditation allows one to function in the astral realms.

Again I saw the colors of the astral realm and the Yellow and Green surrounded in a ball of the Blue and Red. This symbolized the environment and the Earth's body surrounding my body and world. Blue radiates and Red condenses, as Yellow radiates and Green condenses. Time radiates as space condenses. The boundary is permeable and there is exchange in a manner where the external energies and the internal energies interact and yet remain themselves: the boundary remains in place, but energetic and informational Chi is transferred and exchanged. I had several visuals indicating that this is a three way exchange. Perhaps it is input, output, and a continual tension or balancing force which remains in place and yet is dynamic.

There is another image present of a yellow/green above and blue/red below. These are pixelated and racing with vibratory energy. A ball of yellow surrounding green, though both colors existed within and at the boundary and they penetrate below into the blue/red sea, which causes a spray of blue-red droplets to emerge up into the Green/yellow realm. The boundary ripples and the intruding energies and expelled energies are absorbed. This is a good image for the act of breathing, but also symbolic of all data exchanges.

I felt extreme gratitude to the Devi for the gift of a rainbow crystal flower. I received this at a time when I could have made a bad choice with my innate romantic desire. The Devi replied with superb timing and with knowledge of my innermost thoughts. My inner fantasy of the flower was so limited compared to what she offered me visually at that turning point in my life. The Devi has teased me several times and thus brought a longing for the spiritual journey which is much stronger than any worldly desire. The Devi is the Cosmos and perhaps a reflection in my Consciousness, and yet there is the quality of independent sentience in the Cosmos which is seen in synchronicity. **Watching for and following synchronicity is personified as listening to a guardian angel and beside keeping me on the right path, it instills a deep longing, a passion to experience and know the magical treasures of the Devi, the living Cosmos, and also the transcendental personalities who honor me through their interaction.**

Commentary 05:

I cannot write what I experience truthfully and use my mental filters of interpretation to modify my experience. Like my dreams, I do not have a conscious creative intent controlling synchronicities. They are very personal and know me intimately. In this case, I had a fantasy of offering a woman an astral turquoise rose in shared dreaming and at the moment of personal crisis, or perhaps at a possible pivot point within my actions in life, there appears in my mind's eye the Blue Devi and she shows me her large multicolored eyes, enticing me with her celestial beauty, then offers me a crystalline lotus flower, much more sublime than what I had a fantasy of doing.

To imagine that some part of me is superconscious enough to create this vision is very logical, but is not what the experience felt like. Many synchronicities, that are as intimately personal as this experience was, would imply I possess a kind of super Psi power controlling external circumstance, but I don't think that is true. I am not claiming either that the Blue Devi is a Non-Human Intelligence operating in the astral realm and interacting with me as a Guide, nor that I have vast Psi ability which far transcend my reasoning mind. I am reporting experiences which defy humanity's current world view's ability to analyze and explain. The Cosmos which we experience is a vast mystery and we must honestly discuss our actual experiential perceptions to learn and grow.

Session 0065:

Bindu Kala Nada Vak: Out-Breath Bin, In-Breath Do, Out-Breath Kah, In-Breath Lah, Out-Breath Nah, In-Breath Dah, Out-Breath Vach, In-Breath Silent (with a slight lingering and fading Ha sound).

Bindu is a point as in a Plank Quanta, Kala is time, Nada is Resonance, and Vak is the Word. I had trouble with the order to chant in and sometimes I mixed them up. One thing in meditation is to never have self-judgment, just do it. Sometimes there is a natural shift and sometimes a temporary shift which is conveying information. There is no reason to try and determine if the information is from an external source or from one's own mind, as meditation is a non-dual experience: all one knows is what is witnessed within one's awareness.

The visual started with a yellow green field where the waves of green were vertical and vibrating intensely, forming vertical bands. I then saw a plate and a fork, implying that we consume energy/information from our environment. I felt the grounding of my awareness in the lower Dan Tien and a sort of falling into the astral. Then I saw a blue-red field of energy and the red energy was vibrating horizontally and forming bands, waves, or ripples. I had the sensation of stroking or petting the energy field with the breathing of the mantra, as if each out-breath caressed my energy body and involved an energy exchange between the vertical and the horizontal within.

I kept feeling grounded in the lower center, which is life's vital energy, but it was not physical and more of a stability while floating in the astral. I sensed a counter-top, followed by a diving board, and then followed by a diving platform surrounded by a lake, the kind one would swim to and then dive off of. This was followed by a toilet flushing and the water being sucked down. There were black particles in the water, but not waste, and there was nothing gross sensed in the image. Then I was looking down into a tornado, as if I was above and in the calm eye of the storm and swirling power was roaring below. All these images imply that there is vast power in the astral realm or at the Plank scale which is not felt in our daily existence, but is immensely powerful. We are swimming in a lake of energy, diving into it with each in breath, and releasing old energy with each out breath.

Then Vajra entered the chant, this was understood to be both a thunderbolt and a diamond. Here it represented the lightning bolt of plasma discharge. When Bindu, a Plank Quanta, and Kala, the dimensions of time meet in a phenomenal explosion of power which resonates and forms the standing wave of energy or matter. Nada is resonance, the emissive vibratory power which ripples out, but forms constructive interference and thereby the standing waves of energy and matter. Nada is the empowerment of Kundalini, the female force which arises or increases awareness to higher dimensional perception. Like a coiled rattlesnake striking, there are spiraling bursts of energy emitted, virtual particles jump out of the void and are reabsorbed. This is the nature of all of reality! Thoughts jump forth and then dissolve, bodies are born and die, emotions arise and fade away. Everything is wave like: created, sustained, and destroyed.

The next set of images involved the will to sacrifice one's self for the safety or good of a child. This was followed by a birthday celebration, as if to reference the passing on of the torch of life. The words 'You're all set.' came into my mind and it seemed to imply that I am ready for whatever comes next. Then I saw an eye, somewhat stylized as the all-seeing Egyptian eye (of Ra or of Horus). It represents a protective element to the Cosmos that operates at all levels. There is something that drives Consciousness to more perceptive levels and even though personal lives may encounter tragedies, the inner spirit is intensified and refined. I then saw a corridor down a long walkway to a door and sensed that it represented life and we all journey toward a door into the unknown.

This was followed by patterns of flowers, as if kaleidoscopic and as if fractal mandalas. Some were artistic as if created of material mediums and others were of the detail and richness of real flowers. These were beautiful and the message is apparent to enjoy beauty and that the Cosmos spends a good deal of design energy in creating beauty. For all the alternative reasons that science may propose, there appears to be a relational element between humanity and the environment which is facilitated by beauty. **Remember to live with enough lucidity and sensory presence to experience the beauty.**

Session 0066:

Bindu Nada Shabda Hum: Out-Breath Bin, In-Breath Due, Out-Breath Nah, In-Breath Dah, Out-Breath Shab, In-Breath Dah, Out-Breath Hum, In-Breath Mmm (a subtle continuance into silence)

The words refer to a Point, Resonance, Sound, Remembrance (Empowers previous energy): therefore there was a theme, but the order of the words kept changing naturally. The first image was of a large trilobite fossil in a rock and then it was under water and fish were swimming above it. A sense of evolution, the progression of life's journey. Trilobites were one of the longest lasting species of their level of complexity and were in the ocean when fish first evolved. Therefore I believe humans must also evolve if we are to become a long lasting species. I embraced exploring the order of the words, being fluid to seek meaning.

Om Shabda Vajra Hum:
   So returning to Om and having the essence of life in the mantra and then Bindu Nada casting out Vajra: Thunder and Lightning. This is a flash that illuminates and wakes someone up to a higher dimensionality within the subtlety of life. Then I briefly saw a tire and a speed bump and understood that there is resistance to motion and everything moving is limited by what it encounters. Then I saw the inner lightning as a spinning rod which bulged in the center and as it spiraled and moved it shrank. Lightning seems to be a vertical blast down, but I understand energy is flowing up from the Earth, and the idea that the shaft of lightning contains a rotating momentum is intriguing. I have no way to verify this. The aspect of vajra is related to the sudden expelling of energy when two polarities meet.

Om Kali Vajra Hum:
   Adding Kali, the Goddess of time and transformation, came naturally as the next evolution. The resonance of the mantras implies that all touching is sacred and involves a transfer of energy. Touch can facilitate healing transformation. Touch can also be awakening, like a flash of lightning revealing what is hidden in the dark and a clap of thunder startling one to the core and bringing one fully into the present. The sacred touch of Spirit connects the Earth energy to the sky; to the Sun and Moon and to the Milky Way. Human perception makes the bridge between the Earth and the celestial realms. **A healthy human**

has the desire to be kind, to heal others, to give others meaningful gifts, and to be helpful in whatever capacity is possible. I hope my poetry of this text brings brief flashes of realizations to the reader's personal journey which are unique to their nature.

There is often in the process of meditation a pause where one is barely breathing and where the head may droop. Breathing actually slows and one's internal state when one maintains awareness is of floating or drifting in vast astral space. Maintaining awareness and lucid Consciousness requires application of a strong intent, a will to be present in experience. The image of jumping up against gravity and being pulled back down reflects breathing and in deep meditation it is effortless because the sea of fluctuating spatial curvature is breathing one's body. The sense of time changes and one breaths very slow and deep. Thoughts become distractions which cause the leaking of awareness away from being present and perceiving what transpires in the astral space. Staying conscious in meditation is very intense and sensual, blissful and ecstatic, and these feeling satisfy a human need and make one more whole and more peaceful in one's daily life.

Session 0067:

Aum Shakti Sivaya: Out-Breath Ahh, In-Breath uMmm (fading to silence), Out-Breath Shock, In-Breath Tee, Out-Breath Shee, In-Breath Vai, Out-Breath Yah, In-Breath Silence.

The image started with a blue faced woman with exotic features, with a stern and penetrating appearance. This was followed by the statement, 'What exactly is the guarded door, when everything I like is different?' The feeling of this is that the ordinary limitations of a human do not apply to one who has a deep fascination and takes pleasure in the astral realms and in searching out the deepest meanings of life, which will not be properly represented by language as it exists at this time.

Then a blue-red field of energy opened a round portal to look out at a green-yellow scene which was similar to tree covered mountainous land with a valley between the round hills. This was as if looking out of a cave at a natural scene. **This implied that the body-mind vessel is like a cave, but more like a pit, well, or depression; but one can use intent to gaze out at the Sentient Mystery of the Cosmos.** This is implying that Consciousness itself is one polarity and the Cosmos is the other, as if being in a body is to be embedded within the Cosmos and to require personal power to see out of with clarity in order to know the Cosmos which is a Sentient Mystery. If one's being is like a cave or depression in the matrix of the Sentient Mystery, then if it is full of junk on a physical, emotional, or mental level, then one will not be able to experience the Cosmos as it is. One's accumulated junk obscures one's vision and limits one's journey.

At this point I was intent to turn the light of my Consciousness around, meaning to focus on my own source which is the experiencer. I then encountered a guardian at the door of perception. The guardian could appear fierce and defiant, or sweet and wise. It all depended upon my own level of fear and also my intent. To sink into one's own consciousness as a focus can be terrifying or blissful, depending on one's nature. **Therefore the guardians to the inner most essence are the reflection of one's own being and how compassionately loving one is.** From a spatial perspective the essence descended from the head, the ghost cave of mental activity, to the heart, the flower of emotional majesty, to the pit of the abdomen, the center of gravity of the body. From when we lived on the umbilical cord during the forming of our body until death, the essence of our quantum connection is the center of gravity and it implies we are not separate, but in continual relationship with our environment. Thus there is our essence in relationship to the Sentient Mystery of the Cosmos. This implies that knowing one's true essence will equate to knowing the essence of the Cosmos.

Session 0068:

Aum Kali Padme Hum: Out-Breath Awe or Ahh, In-Breath Mmm fading to silence, Out-Breath Kah, In-Breath Lee, Out-Breath Paud, In-Breath Ma, Out-Breath Hoom, In-Breath Silence.

The Queen Devi's presence as the tone of inquiry became present and the message was to be aware of how gender and natural sexual qualities influence one's perception. In my case I refer to the Queen Devi as feminine and that is how I perceive her, but there is no real way for me to qualify this and someone could just as easily sense the King Deva, a masculine presence. As stated in the introduction, there is no concern about whether the deity has material existence as in occupying an external body, or is an astral individual sentience, or a dream form within my psyche. What followed was an image of a mother with a child on a tricycle, teaching and protecting the child. Thus, there is the implication that any superior celestial being which is teaching and protecting would be sensed as maternal in my unique mind, but might be paternal energy for someone else.

This was followed by the astral reference to lost humans with power and their descent into unconsciousness. The true celestial being, while having power to control and manipulate, cannot transfer true wisdom through power. All that a teacher or guide can do is to point out the way. Everyone is unique and must learn the lessons of life for themselves. One cannot be given spiritual power, it is inherent in one's essential nature, but lies sleeping. The teacher can display the wisdom to the extent that the pupil can grasp it, but often there are beginning steps which must proceed a more advanced level of awakening. Complete awakening is a lyrical myth of storytelling, there is always more the Cosmos can offer one who is open to receive. As in language and mathematics, one must comprehend the basics before being able to consider advanced scholarly dissertations, therefore spiritual wisdom, which is the real behind all symbolism, must be grasped as living experience, thus the richness of a life is gained with meditation.

Then the image was of a giant statue of a being, a teacher or god representation. This was followed by standing before a giant stone lion and due to the size of it, I could not tell if a deity was riding it, but assumed that Durga, the goddess as protector, was being shown. Such statues assure some passage of wisdom down numerous generations and reveal that the ancients had concepts which were important enough to them to set in stone. Statues and images are fluid and non-linear teachings which allow each experiencer to gain direct wisdom.

Then I saw a human mouth with large sensual lips and frightening teeth. This was paradoxical, as if the Sweet Blue Devi and the Wild Blue Devi were actually one being. We all contain the ability to express ourselves in different ways. Durga is the protector of the universe and therefore is the mother of all the beings in the universe, while also is one of the most powerful and fierce warriors. Some will love her and some will fear her depending on their relationship to spiritual life.

Then in pixelated form I saw a disc shaped craft with windows along the flat ring between the top and the bottom. This was followed by the wisdom that true communication is a collaboration. Both sides must be open to listen and to share honestly. **Listening is an art and the essence must be to really hear what is said as it is intended, rather than searching out points to reply for one's own opinion.** Then the question was raised to my contemplating mind, "Who buys the tickets?" In other words, what are the two sides in a communication and or collaboration offering. Whether material advanced beings, astral beings, or transcendental celestial beings, one must enter into communication: the collaboration of shared dialog toward wisdom, must be accompanied by an offering. One must offer time with complete attention and the energy to maintain intent. One is to consider what service they may offer in the ongoing energy of the communication, not just what they are to receive.

Then the Sweet Blue Devi became present and I saw a flock of birds flying in formation. When one encounters any sentient being, one must consider that the sentient being is in relationship with others. When one communicates wisdom to a person, if that person gains insight, they will share the communication. This was followed by the internal blue energy weaving with red energy, the two geometries interacting with dynamic tension and the resultant of a blue pearl arising, followed by a red pearl. The entwining dance of two points of view are like a fabric within which standing waves rise up where they are connected. The cosmic essence and the human essence, differentiated and yet entwined in a being. This was followed by the blue-red fabric fading to almost black, then white orbs forming patterns with symbolic meanings to point the way. **Symbols, such as words, or any notation or art, can only point at something, for the truth has a rich and complex nature which can be represented by symbols, but can only be known through experience.** Real life is so amazingly complex and yet so elegantly refined that no symbolic reflection can communicate it. We are each a miracle.

Session 0069:

Aum Kali Durga Hum: Out-Breath Awe or Ahh, In-Breath uMmm fading to silence, Out-Breath Kah, In-Breath Lee, Out-Breath Der, In-Breath Gah, Out-Breath Hoom, In-Breath Silence.

   The first astral image was of a peacock feather display. This was followed by the image of the TicTac UFO video screen and I got the impression this was a theater in the sky, showing off like a peacock. Then I saw a long narrow lake with manmade sides along the base of a mountain and then continuing out into the countryside. After first seeing it, when I was viewing it from above as a drone would see it, I followed it and it stretched for many miles. I then saw a huge rocket and the message was, 'I am tired of rockets and hiding secrets from spies'. All together this amounts to a call to end the charade and allow humanity to get off the planet (which chemical rockets cannot accomplish). Star Trek is our future, but the Cosmos is filled with amazing advanced cultures far superior to current humanity and yet we can be the cutting edge of evolution if we stop sabotaging ourselves.
   I then saw a very colorful mandala which transformed into a whirlwind and then the Sweet Blue Devi's face. Her blue face was incredibly beautiful and I thought of kissing and it faded. I then saw a shell of metal armor around a body and then it fit closer as if it became worn. This was followed by a shirt with blue and white horizontal stripes, but presented the idea that clothes were a type of armor and also it related to the peacocks display. At that point I realize that the beautiful Devi's face may just be a mental projection which appeared like a human face, but was unlikely to be this blue being's true form. Perhaps the image was like an avatar. Did it intend to cause desire to arise in me or was it innocence just trying to be beautiful?
   I was led to contemplate humanity and the changes which cataclysms have had upon us. The example of the Mount Toba super-volcano eruption which was around seventy-four thousand years ago and reduced the human population to perhaps less than ten thousand people; though it is hard to say the exact number, such genetic bottlenecks have occurred. The recovery and changes to the environment must have been profound, resulting in extreme changes to the human genome. Then there was the Younger Dryas comet and solar storm around twelve thousand nine hundred years ago which caused the flood, the oceans rising perhaps as much as a hundred and fifty meters and a thousand

years of cold. Again coastal humanity was wiped out and the change in environment must have changed the human genome profoundly.

My visioning also included the bee hive which we have and which swarmed. The worker bees who live from fifteen to forty days in the warm seasons would be encountering different flowers. Then changes in the hive from a box being harvested would also present a change. If our hive split, then the new generation will have a completely different environment. It is interesting to consider the changes to humanity with natural geologic changes, but now humans are mutating from chemicals and use of electronics. The genetic change in humans is speeding up and the climate disaster could result in the surviving portion of humanity being quite different than humans today. If one considers the change in human body size due to modern nutrition from a thousand years ago, the change is geologically extremely rapid. The question becomes: can humanity gain enough awareness to direct our changes into becoming more conscious beings.

I then got the sense of not wanting to be caged, physically or mentally. **There is an inherent urge within humanity to be free.** Perhaps we will create the technology to be free to explore the solar system and then the stars. Perhaps we will be able to free our minds of illusions and claim our inherently psychic nature. I then saw a Yellow Warrior Devi, perhaps a Durga image. At first just presence, very hard to see, blending into the astral background. Then She had a frightfully powerful look and when I recoiled she laughed and assumed a sweet form, I did not fear, but was taken aback and cautious. I got the sense of a very advanced world.

Then a beautiful turquoise orb appeared and the Queen Devi looked on. This was followed by a small cylinder, perhaps a ring for a longer finger. Its background was in yellow with tan and orange shades and very distinct and clear turquoise streaks surrounded in black. It was glossy. It was very aesthetically pleasing and the colors were perfectly balanced and yet had a natural aspect. I contemplated the nature of being and of the essence consciousness and the aspect of true creativity and the ability to make choices which are the defining characteristics of sentient beings. **Sentient beings are twofold, possessing awareness, receptivity, but also possessing an active will, intent, guided by awareness.** The ability to be creative is one of the most essential faculties for humans to continue evolving through the hard times.

Finally I got traditional images of Kali wearing sculls as jewelry (time catches all, she will wear your skull and mine as well) and Durga with powerful weapons. I could not see her clearly, but her Warrior nature was apparent. The statement, 'It is all starting to go down!' I wondered if it was a battle for Earth or for human souls. I wondered if it was a battle to allow humanity to know their true history, which would give us a real perspective to live from. I wondered how much humans were helped in the past to survive the catastrophes and how the ancient myths and legends were descriptions of the truth, slightly deformed by passing down through the ages. Are Durga and Kali to emerge again and destroy the demons that are ravaging Mother Earth?

Session 0070:

Aham Sauh: Out-Breath Ah, In-Breath Hum, Out-Breath Sow, In-Breath hhh (Fading to silence).

The first image was of a camera pointed at me. Then the Queen Devi's face very close up, mostly her right eye. They are watching me, us. I say they because at the consciousness level of the Queen Devi, there is not the personal ego due to sharing everything in a telepathic collective. Humans tend to beg their personally chosen Goddess or God for things, but it is time for a shift of energy, or perhaps I should say energy is shifting and will not be denied. It is time to serve the Goddess or God which one personifies. **As a shower cleans one's body, so will the telepathic revealing of every thought and feeling wash our minds.** The grace that will pour down will not judge one's state, but will demand we clean up our act. There is no hiding from higher consciousness.

The Queen Devi's face morphed into a horse scull and then presented me with visions of a mouth devouring. Her telepathic vision and her photographic memory allow her to know us better than we know ourselves. Then a question was put forth to me, "Do you trust the mature lady?". She, the Devi Queen, has the inside scoop on all we do, but can we admit to ourselves what she sees and refine our intent until we can trust her enough to let down our guard and open communication? **We might not want to hear what the Goddess has to say, but it will definitely do us good to accept the truth and work from there.**

At this moment in meditation I also perceived many panels, with cryptic data, as if symbolic of sets of data, which were shuffling about to find intertwining patterns. The Queen Devi does not live in our world view and cannot understand the paradigm from which it is constructed. Unlike transparent telepathic beings such as the Queen Devi, who have individuality and bodies, but can overcome illusions and function as consciousness, every human lives in our own little parallel world. We lack a true consensus reality and what little consensus reality our ancestors shared, humans today are losing the cohesiveness of those shared beliefs. Since society is filled with oligarchies who manipulate lies for control and power, most humans have lost faith in any particular consensus reality.

After settling into the void of deep meditation, which is bliss and pure being, but does not contain differentiation and is without sequential time, always seeming like a moment, like a deep sleep, in which I remain conscious, I emerged in the astral to see a small figure clocked in black, almost comical, walking up the driveway of a neighbor's house in suburbia. Her imagery is ironic and somewhat comical, as if it is part play or done for enjoyment as well as for teaching. The Queen Devi moves through our reality as if a little ninja spy, snooping in our minds, hoping to help us break out of our mental delusions. Do not be fooled into thinking it is about someone else, it is every single one of us. **She watches and subtly interacts with every human, but most shut out her grace.**

This was followed by a horse carrying baskets, symbolizing us humans carrying the baggage of countless things and I recalled her showing me a horse scull: we cannot carry stuff with us when we die. When we lose our body, we lose our language and so lose our belief in words, our mythology. Our human form, our body-mind vessels are containers of the light of consciousness and that light spills out in sensory experience. We form our world by a power of our consciousness. Every animal and plant has a different world view. The human view is not real, it is a diminished reflection of the real, but this mirror of our beings is clouded by our false ideas. The Queen Devi and her associates offers us freedom from our illusions, from the distortions which beliefs place upon our reflection. When we clean our minds of delusions, the Queen Devi can interact to a greater degree and we can be of service to each other as human community, taking our first steps out of our collective confusion about the nature of these sacred incarnations which we are experiencing.

Session 0071:

OM Kali Krishna Hum: Out-Breath Ohh, In-Breath Mmm (fading to silence), Out-Breath Kah, In-Breath Lee, Out-Breath Kree, In-Breath Shahna, Out-Breath Hum, In-Breath silence.

We went to a talk by a modern guru, which was OK, but nothing deep was said verbally. He had people take children from the auditorium and the lights dimmed as if a movie would start. He then led 800 people in a movement exercise for neck and shoulder stress relief, then had everyone close their eyes. He did the sensing exercise (Feel your feet relax, Feel you ankles relax, Feel you calves relax, ... up through the whole body). Then in silence he had people sense the walls of the auditorium, though it was completely dark. This was interesting as I could easily visualize the space, almost as if seeing or sensing the walls. Then we were to sense the ceiling above us. These were good exercises in using second sight.

While no mention of mantra was brought up, I used mantra the whole time. I have been working since the last meditation on combining Kali and Krishna, since they are equated as female and male forms of time, all attractive (time), and are both warriors destroying the enemies of life. The Sweet Blue Devi's face appeared followed by a male form of the face, which I shall term Blue Deva. Blue Deva was peaceful and calm. Then the feminine blue face reappeared very clear and she had her eyes closed and appeared blissful. She seemed to be soaking in the energy. Then her face faded and the Queen Devi appeared briefly. Then the sweet Blue Devi's face reappeared. It seemed like the faces were morphing dream images, but then I got the mental impression that the Queen Devi watches through the Blue Devi's being.

I cannot say if there is any physical reality to these beings, or if they are just in my mind. What I can say is that they were blissful in the presence of so many humans sitting together in peace and silence. **I felt like this was a message that such group meditations were the path for a positive human future: for peace on Earth and goodwill among all people.** I live in a rural setting at this time, but have facilitated group meditations in the past. I am not sure how to facilitate this and the famous Guru character we had seen was teaching at a level far below what anyone can access with mantra meditation, but then that was a general admission show. I do not follow human gurus. The true gurus are the transcendental beings and my mind personifies them as Goddesses and Gods, while knowing the totality of creation rests in the ultimate-supreme, and we all have a relationship with that indescribable sentience.

Session 0072:

Aum Kali Radhe Hum: Out-Breath Ahh, In-Breath uMmm, Out-Breath Kah, In-Breath Lee, Out-Breath Rahd, In-Breath Hey, Out-Breath Hum, In-Breath Silence.

   Well we had the floor being repaired with electric saws, hammers, and the workers had on loud modern country music. I was on the porch with the dog, but I figured why not meditate. One should not let conditions of one's environment prevent meditation. In this condition what arose was a poem, one line at a time:

We love the flower.
Seeds are precious.
The temporary nature
of our lives challenges us.

Fascinated with babies.
Troubled by the dying.
Love songs always popular
as fantasy hypnotizes.

Sleep demands we submit.
Seasons cycle past our windows.
Every moon waxes and wanes
as we rush through the visit:

Pause and Meditate!

Session 0073:

Aum Kali Radhe Hum: Out-Breath Ahh, In-Breath uMmm, Out-Breath Kah, In-Breath Lee, Out-Breath Rahd, In-Breath Hey, Out-Breath Hum, In-Breath Silence.

    Love endures aging. Love transcends time. The quantum string connection created through sex is a silver cord channel which remains forever. Sexual attraction is a reflection of our sense of Unity and our desire to know the bliss and ecstasy of spiritual Unity. From the higher dimensions our minds are naked. There is vulnerability in opening oneself to love and yet with all humility we stand beckoning the sacred and divine presence. **My bodily form is filled with vibration as I sense the feminine sentience of the Cosmos looking in on me.** The Cosmos and the situations falling from the future often have total power and control. I accept the new adventures life presents to me. I am not worthy, but I am in need, and therefore I offer myself to a new path whenever I can see the divine guidance to do so.

    I get the visual of a green backpack where I have protected goods. Am I ready to reveal my baggage and deal with it. Can I stand before the sacred presence of brilliant Consciousness and see what truly is? The table of offerings that was imagined as all rose flowers is protected by thorns. If one does not want the inner baggage to go rotten and fester and be revealed as offensive, then one must take it out into awareness and purify it. There is no shame in the past which is admitted and renounced. **Meditation is purifying work and is much more efficient at freeing one from the past than anything the thinking mind could do.** The resonance of the mantra vibrates one and all the baggage is shaken off and falls away. One becomes free to be a compassionate and loving being by choosing to go forward in the truth of one's cosmos, the limited personal reality one knows, which is as it is, and with the light of Conscious awareness, choosing one's path to expand one's world view.

    In the vision of lumber being used to remodel a house I continually see the option of using Meditation to remodel my self and my life. Time and the changes falling from the future into our life are sometimes unexpected and sometimes bring forth powerful emotions. **The Sentient Mystery of the Cosmos is cultivating our Consciousness and intensifying our awareness, which is our true being as seen in meditation.** This awareness of our essence as the Consciousness perceiving is coupled with our Spirit making choices and transcends our personality and worldly self-image. The Mystery of the Cosmos Spirit nurtures our essence, our personal conscious spirit.

If one sees a score of music and all those notes on the page, and one can read it and play it, it takes on a different significance when listened to. The entire piece of music has a vibration which touches deeper than the mind can think about. When a song holds magic for a person, there is an aesthetic pleasure which is naturally distilled in the experiential listening and which touches one's essence in indescribable ways. Meditation is like that at a higher level and is a type of love which nurtures the true essence of one's being. Gradually as one meditates for daily brief pauses in one's life and experiences one's own true nature, one goes forth living life with more awareness, feeling more alive, and ready to engage whatever one must to be true to one's compassionate and loving self.

Session 0074:

Sauh: Out-Breath Sau, In-Breath uHhhh (fading to silence).

 I kept slipping into the void and my head would bob and I would become aware of myself meditating. The mantra was continuous, my awareness was slipping into the state where nothing is distinguished. This is why several ancients texts state that only the changes of interactions with the Perceived stimulates awareness into being or only the Cosmos awakens consciousness, sustains consciousness, and reabsorbs consciousness. Without the changes of life, consciousness would not be nurtured to expand.
 I became aware of a key question while seeing what arises in the mind, that question being, 'Why these specific things'? What has recently passed in our life experience is one factor, but does not account for all that arises. What do we bring up out of past memory? What do we dream at night? In all cases our recent life experiences and some deeper past experiences do play a role, but there are other thoughts and memories which arise suddenly and without precedence. There is a mechanism and it is not random. **In some cases a sentience to the order and impact of what arises becomes apparent.** An external Consciousness would also be internal if we are aware of it in our Consciousness, making the internal and external duality of no purport. All that arises is either a reflection of our accumulated and assembled being (the past pushing on us) or the changes we encounter in the Mystery of our life line (the future pulling on us, attracting us into waiting potentials).
 Then I saw a set of carts hitched together and going by. The first one was fur lined for comfort and the last one had lumber, which references the recent meditation where it represented remodeling one's personality. Therefore, I get the impression that maintaining comfort is secondary to the need to embrace change. Remodeling one's home includes an uncomfortable period of transition, but then, if done with wisdom, it is worth it and is a more comfortable and functional space. So it must be with the personality, the who we are in the world.
 Next, amid dipping into the void and having my head bob and coming back into awareness, I thought of my wife Beth. There is a paradox to the idea we are all one, that is that we each have a unique spirit will and have assembled unique experiences from our lives to be who we presently are. **In a relationship one must separate the placing of one's own filters of seeing the person in a specific way from**

honoring who they really are. Balancing the give and take of two wills, two intents, is indeed a life skill which one must refine into an art form in order to live harmoniously. These skills need to refine all our relations. It does not mean a battle of wills, but instead a deeper seeing of the duality of other in the relationship of together. All humans are together and we need to see each other realistically as opposed to by our personal mental ideas. Awareness and acceptance of what is provides the first step in creating the harmony which creates a building resonance between nodes of our relationships.

Finally I saw a giant evergreen tree with activity and stuff under it. It was shaped as an equilateral triangle pointing up, which is the symbol for masculinity. Yet, under the ground, at the roots supporting it would be a triangle pointing down, which represents feminine energy, which supports the tree of life. There is a great need to embrace the energy of nurturing and having that energy replace the battle of wills. There is a gentle power in nurturing others which overcomes the striving of wills. There is a greater power in supporting someone to become their unique self, than in making others conform to one's own ideas of them. This does not imply being used or condoning destructive behavior, but instead finding ways to nurture the root compassionate and loving person which every human is capable of being. Life is complex and people are complex, but true nurturing can be a way of life guided by embodying compassionate and loving feeling which transcends all ideas and beliefs.

Session 0075:

Radhe Radha Radharani: Out-Breath Ra(h)d, In-Breath (d)Hey, Out-Breath Ra(h)d, In-Breath (d)Ha(h), Out-Breath Ra(h)d, In-Breath (d)Ha(h), Out-Breath Ra(h), In-Breath Knee.

'Children do not grow through mental interaction, but rather through experiential interaction.' Adults are like this also, they act according to what they see and experience, sometimes even contrary to what the mind states logically. After these words came a visual of the Blue Devi, the first with a set of white orbs circling her head in a dance, like a halo which was celebrating. **The emotions of love, very human and also very divine, might not always seem logical, but the true experience of the human journey is 'we become enraptured in love'.** If it is a fall from logic or from a solitary life, it is the practical source of fulfillment of our human journey and in relationship we spiritually transcend beyond our self-centered personality and become more.

The next visual was very spatial of a large stone room, cathedral-like with stone coffins The Blue Devi's face was very close and her eyes were peering at me, then she became hidden. A male Blue Deva appeared and also faded. There was emptiness without the living presence, regardless of the gender of one's devotion. Then a young Golden Devi face appeared, but it aged and the skin became loose and the color changed until it became the Wild Blue Devi, fierce and mocking, like the erosion of time which consumes everything. This is the nature of the Mystery which we as Consciousness are embedded within.

Then the words which arose were, 'You are large and extraordinary in this situation.' and I knew it was not speaking to me personally, but to humanity. Humans have extraordinary Consciousness which may witness a lifetime from a higher perspective, as a journey. The transformations lose their frightening nature and one finds peace as the Consciousness perceiving the dance of time; of the changes falling from the future though the hourglass of one's life and depositing the sands of the past forever.

Then I saw an old gray wooden barn with a single window in the center of its side which had four panes of glass. I entered the barn and it was dark except for a single candle which seemed to be dwarfed in the large space. Then I could vaguely make out the Golden Devi, a very old soul with a young face. I got the impression that what the mind conceives of as impossible is not always impossible and that phenomenal predictions might come true. The Golden Devi illuminated by the candle is like the illumination of the mind: a very dim reflection of a miraculous multidimensional life force. When one re-associates their being to the essence Consciousness, the true experiencer, then the Golden Goddess is revealed dancing in the sunlight in glory. The world view that we are conditioned into is like an old barn, empty and although seeming structurally sound the foundation is fading and it is soon to collapse.

Then the Devi's words are, 'When you go up there with your family, there are multiple things which can happen.' I understood up there to imply as a being living from Consciousness and in the presence of the Celestial Devi-s and Deva-s. They are our family and also our Ancestors are our family, as well as all our relations in life. One's level of Compassionate Love determines how one it treated, not as reward or punishment, but as what level one can embody. **You cannot teach calculus to someone who cannot comprehend algebra.** What one can experience and also what one's mind can assimilate for one to use in decision making must grow from where one is at. One is called to be humble enough to see the truth of where one is at, because from there one may grow.

Then the next words of the Devi were, 'After that I was lost for a few years with everybody, everyone, looking in.' Again I do not take these words as personal, when we first 'Go up there' into a higher state of Consciousness and actually experience a higher state of awareness, we lose the grounding of living in the old gray barn of our conditioned belief system. Then we must work hard for years to sort out all the implications and learn the foundational wisdom which can create a new home, a new world view. The words which followed were, 'If given back a completely clear memory of a time when you were young, you will still view it from your current point of view.' This exemplifies that our world view, our limited paradigm of reality, is the world we live in. **The Sacred Mystery which Consciousness experiences is beyond all world views.** The symbolic reflections of the mind which color experience are a very limited reflection of what is.

The next phrase was, 'Lands, each person has a realm, and you drink the blood of the... [realm, lands]'. The Wild Devi energy is here, being graphic in telling us that we each live in our own parallel universe, our own paradigm built upon the paradigm of the culture and times we live in, and we drink from what we believe. Every belief is a mythology, symbolic words built into a lesser dimensional description of the glorious, sacred, and divine Mystery of the Cosmos. I see the Queen Devi's right eye so close that it fills my vision, like a black mirror upon which my image of myself, my limited reflection of who I am, shimmers and then she closes her all seeing, all knowing eye, and I am floating in the void. The Celestials of the higher Spiritual Sky and our essence Consciousness when freed of the filters of a mythology of belief become experiential. The void becomes filled with dancing blue-red energy which is transmuted to green-yellow: meaning this is how we get unstuck on ourselves and embrace relationship which is Unity, the Way of Love.

Next I see brilliant red seeds, which were smooth and shiny, followed by a vision of a very advanced technological vast space, like the inside of a metal cavern. The lucid astral (dream) tells me, 'You are going to need it like this.'; meaning humanity will need technology to survive. The red seeds are the most brilliant humans who will figure out aspects of the Mystery which are waiting for us to discover so that we can prosper. I am told these brilliant red seeds are those who know mantra and are chosen by their natural ability to envision what no one yet knows and bring it into our paradigm.

I see a stone hill and underground is a home, completely hidden. I am told, 'We know suffering and we are watching.' I see the Queen Devi. Nothing which humanity does is hidden from her gaze. Everyone of a higher Consciousness is looking in on humanities foolishness and outdated, false belief paradigms. A new future waits for Humanity, the challenge is for us to embrace it.

Session 0076:

Aum Kali Ma Krishna Hum: Out-Breath Aum, In-Breath Mmm (fading), Out-Breath Kah, In-Breath Lee, Out-Breath Ma, In-Breath Hhh (fading), Out-Breath Kree, In-Breath Shnah, Out-Breath Hum, In-Breath Mmm (fading).

    I see thumbs and the one to the left is clear. Then I sense some of the chant being more on the right side. The thought words seemed to pan differently. Then the Mmmm which was rising was centered. A message arose, 'I think this is an ancient key.' It seemed spoken in the dream space rather than being a thought I was having. This mantra is very powerful and I sensed a warning that this should be done by emotionally stable individuals and not taken lightly. Kali and Krishna were both Warriors. They Killed those who were on errant pathways and also creatures with demonic mentality. They both say, 'I am time'.

    I then found myself in a library which was the archives of time. I saw an inverted equilateral triangle (symbol of the feminine trinity of energies) in the dust at the foot of a bookshelf. I reached down and tried to find it with my hand in the dust, but it disappeared as a mirage. One aspect is that the corners are left, right, and center. I sensed Kree of Krishna opening the central channel of energy within my being and shnah as a rising current of energy. I sensed Kah of Kali as grounded at the base of my seat and Lee as rising energy. The words arose, 'Walk slowly in the Void', which I took to mean move ones awareness slowly up the central channel.

    Karma is like dust collecting on your socks if you walk without shoes upon the unclean floor of false mental beliefs. Karma scurries across the floor of one's life like a mouse seeking the lost crumbs, the illogical cyclic thought loops driven by emotional delusions. One's inner space is one's home, the external dwelling place upon one's visit to Earth. Krishna is pure Consciousness which is at home in Kali Ma, the fierce and controlling energy behind the play of the Cosmos. When Krishna embraces Radha, when Consciousness embraces that which is all attractive, it is said her golden complexion turns to dark sapphire as day turns into night, and all dances fall within Kali, the controlling laws of time. I then see the Sweet Devi, her blue face with her eyes closed, blissful in the Union of meditation. Contained within an inverted glass of perception the Devi appears as the meek Golden Devi, but set free she is the all-powerful Wild Blue Devi.

The red leash of one's body and the limitations of one's incarnation are the Devi's game within which one can find true freedom through embracing life fully. I perceive a Red Deva, a male offering a shelf of books: Consciousness reading the library of time and seeing the hidden aspects of the Devi's play. Hum: one's spiritual heart may open to receive all that falls from the future upon one. I receive words, 'I would not exercise, never!' and I understand this to mean, there is great work to be done, be of service. If one studies a musical instrument, or one's being, the motivation is curiosity and the enjoyment of playing, not the egotistical seeking of fame or fortune. One is continually challenged by learning new music, new aspects of life, and yet one is playful and exploring. Rather than engaging in mental exercises, engage in true contemplation with a deep wondering; seek to find the solutions to the puzzles life presents one with. Avoid the grandiose endeavors driven by one's ego and embrace the compassionate service work which is available in life, the work of one's spiritual heart.

I see the Sweet Blue Devi's face in the distance, looking sad and hallow due to the separation which human Consciousness has from her magnificent living being. Then I see the Queen Devi's left eye close and she is whispering in my ear secrets of life and creation. She is saying in her telepathic communication, 'End your fantasies. Heal your being by opening your spiritual heart. Accept the unfolding Mystery of the Cosmos with absolute Consciousness. Be fully present in your life and be fully present for others. Krishna is your Consciousness, the experiencer, the enjoyer. Kali is all that happens in your personal play of life, the Conscious unfolding of the Cosmos. Your Spirit, the power of your intent, is the Union, where the duality dissolves, and you're completely present and completely transcendental: Completely alive.' This message was not in these exact words, but in a conveyed expression with feeling.

Finally the message of the secret of the Golden Flower, the Golden Lotus, the Golden Devi, echoes in my awareness, "Turn your Light around". The Golden Yellow is the Consciousness in all of nature, in the entire Cosmos, in the Green. The Deep Blue, the Dark Sapphire, is the Consciousness embodied in my form, in my incarnation, the Red thread of mortal life. When Consciousness turns around to its source, its center, its axis, then it finds Union with the Supreme Devi and there is only timeless bliss and ecstasy amid the flowing time: Krishna and Kali, Consciousness and Spirit, occupying ones Spiritual Heart. Aum is the 'Yes' as a verb, it is the thrill of true love being fulfilled in experiential activity, it is the Sacred embracing the Divine and the merging into Union.

Session 0077:

Kali Hum Krishna Hum: Out-Breath Kah, In-Breath Lee, Out-Breath Hoom, In-Breath Mmmm (fading to silence), Out-Breath Kree, In-Breath Shahna, Out-Breath Hoom, In-Breath Mmmm (fading to silence).

As I became aware of my breath, I realized that breathing is time. It is a true cycle of time that Consciousness is bound within. One's awareness and focus affect breathing and breathing can affect one's state of mind. Maintaining the Mantra with the breath brings one to a calm and even breath which changes one's frequency and one enters into the deeper levels of inner space. Soon the astral realm opened and I saw the Queen Devi looking at me from a place that is more still, as a being who's Consciousness is not caught in time the way human Consciousness is. There were no thoughts, this was a set of feelings in the astral dream.

As feelings invited the thought words to encapsulate them in a more limited symbolic form I perceived that the thinking mind had pulled me out of the experience and put me in mental space which can only ruminate about the past. The mind is looking downstream as we travel upon the river of time in which we keep moving upstream. Meditation involves being on the current edge of the here and now, while simultaneously turning one's light of Consciousness around to look upstream, to face the future. **In this process one realizes that the more subtle dimensions fall though Consciousness first and sensory data lags by a very small margin.** Thus, as one goes deeper into the Meditation and one's awareness is fully dedicated to breathing the Mantra, then the finer dimensionality of the unfolding play of manifestation enters one's awareness.

Then the astral image of an old wooden sailing ship on the ocean of time appeared. This was a good image since the momentum of the past is like the wind driving the ship, but the ship has some ability to navigate. At the same time the changes falling from the future into one's life are like the ocean and the changes in weather which necessitate activity to deal with. Then dream words arose, 'What is going on in the rest of the ship?' This can be considered personal, in reference to one's body and the external life conditions affect how one may deal with the changes falling from the future, as well as globally, since all of humanity shares the Earth. One has a responsibility for the shape of one's personal life and also to contribute to the common good in whatever humble way one is called to do so. Good choices and simple acts of compassion can influence the course of the ship and therefore what changes are encountered in the future.

I realized on the in-breath of Hum which is the long and sublime 'Mmmm' fading to silence is facing time forward. If is contrary to entropy. Forward time is that which powers the spirit of life. **The in-breath is the healing breath and should be deep and long for every breath in our life.** Mantra meditation can heal our breathing pattern which will bring healing power to the whole body. 'Kah' is grounding and 'Lee' is energy rising up the central channel of our body to space over the head. Although there is a materialist tendency to associate this with the spinal column, it is not physical, but the energetic power of Consciousness. 'Kree' opens the central channel and 'Shahna' is a spiral unwinding in higher dimensionality as it ascends. These two aspects are said to be female and male counterparts and when used together they amplify each other's energy. The in-breath is the healing and loving power. The out-breath is the grace which allows the in-breath to work.

Finally when one has ascended into higher realms of perception through breathing mantra, one feels telepathically and empathically the web of humanity and the Living Earth and there is great pain and suffering. One is incited to call for compassionate love. One is called to stand up for the innocent and powerless. The Queen Devi watches the drama of humanity and I call to her to intercede, to take action such that the laws of the heavens be applied to the Earth and humanity is brought back into the balance for the love of the future generations. Intention, from dream space and from the mind, is the key in steering the ship of life toward future seas of peace and prosperity.

Session 0078:

Aum Durga Padma Radha Hum: Out-Breath ahhh, In-Breath uMmm, Out-Breath Dur, In-Breath Gah, Out-Breath Pod, In-Breath Mah, Out-Breath Rad, In-Breath Ha, Out-Breath Hum, In-Breath Mmmm (fading to Silence).

    I envision two people starting to climb a mountainside and they are about three meters (ten feet) up and it is already perilous. Durga is a warrioress like Krishna and Radha is a devoted lover. Durga is a protective aspect of the supreme Devi and Radha is the sweet and tender, vulnerable aspect. Padma is a Lotus Flower, a sacred symbol of Shakti, the creatrix of the Cosmos. Aum is one's essence Consciousness residing in Hum, the spiritual heart. Therefore the aspects might seem very different, but they all represent different natures of the one supreme. In this case the vibratory nature of the thought-sounds seemed related and the out-breaths all had the H sound fading to silence, which causes a radiating of the energy invoked.
    I then perceived an oval high rise of great height, as if from a science fiction image. It gave me a feeling of many people trapped away from the natural world, away from the living Cosmos. Red and blue were cycling with green and yellow in my astral vision which washed away the behemoth high rise. **Our inner natural being must have connection to the outer natural world to be healthy.** I then sensed, 'There is another piece.' and it's as if another telepathic message comes to clarify the one received. The oval shape would be immune to winds which would ravage a square building. Having people concentrated in living space could allow for vast natural lands and also land for growing the food they need. If people had easy access to go outside, then they would not be trapped. This is similar to being in our body: we are not trapped in flesh, it is a gift and our freedom remains in our higher senses.
    We are each required by life to conquer our demons, to chew on life's situations and digest what lessons we may glean from the changes imposed upon us. We can feel the wrong paths in our gut and we can remove them by correcting our choices. What are we doing with our precious time? Durga holds a sword of light which illuminates our every thought and deed, cutting through the lies we tell to ourselves so that we might know where we are and grow from the present condition. Radha offers us a Lotus of beauty and blessing if we are willing to

accept it, if we are worthy within our own sense of our real selves, without delusions.

I then perceived seals lounging on ice by a cold sea. They were in their proper environment and although it would be harsh for a human, it was wonderfully comfortable to them. **We each need to find the environment in which we can thrive.** I sensed the two Blue Devi, one sweet and one fierce, skiing in the wake of my life, coming up behind me, watching and reacting to the motion of my life, my mind, and my innermost feelings. I then saw a star pattern and it reformed into a sleek futuristic jet. They are not limited by our sense of what is possible, but they cannot make life choices for us, so they fly behind us, sometimes breaking into our awareness, offering a warning or offering a glimpse of beauty. Will we listen to their directions, avoid the pitfalls or stop to relish the beauty(?) - It is up to us to choose.

Next I envisioned someone trying to pull a prank on someone else and slipping and falling on their back. A red demon roared at the attempted folly. The Devi are tricksters, but not pranksters. They have a sense of humor, sometimes heavy and sometimes light, but they only wish to enhance our conscious awareness. They are not seeking anything for themselves; they are only offering us gifts. Demons seek to gain control and manipulate us, whether they are pranking us into addictions, habitual tendencies, or false concepts of reality. When one tells a lie, to themselves or to others, situations change and they need more lies to continue, until they slip in their own web of deception and fall.

I then saw a white book, it was unknown to humans, but very sacred. I was informed that sometimes a Devi has a way of sneaking into our reality, of operating at a higher frequency and remaining invisible. There is sentience to the Cosmos and that sentient energy influences the changes we encounter in life. **There are synchronicity guiding our way which are very intimately personal.** Beware of what you follow, use the guiding principle of love to judge choices available. It can be very complex, Durga is a warrioress and Radha is a lover. They are examples of the Fierce Blue Devi and the Sweet Blue Devi, but both are aspects of the divine. It is in defending the way of love that a warrior is most powerful and it is in revealing and acting with love that one is most vulnerable: to be fully human we must deal with the changes that fall from the future into our lives with love.

Session 0079:

Meonia: In-Breath Me On Eye, Out-Breath a (as in cat).

    Not a Sanskrit term, but rather from European esoteric tradition. I decided to work with it because it is just vowels and 'm' and 'n'. In Sanskrit one poetic analogy is that vowels are seeds and consonants grow them and clothe them with form (Bija and Yoni). There is also the mantric impression that 'm' is feminine and 'n' is masculine and therefore having both is balanced. The last syllable 'a' is the first character of the alphabet, representing Anuttara, the supreme, the union of the totality beyond words, and so that becomes the exhale. I grew up on mantras with a triplet in-breath, which also orients me in this way. An in-breath can be sensed to have three parts.
    My first impression was the phrase, "Because your dad was looking for you. He asked to see yours." and I felt this to imply our heavenly Father (the living Cosmos) seeking our real being, rather than our constructed and conditioned personality. I felt as I heard the words that yours, a possessive term, implied my whole life, all that I have done, all the creativity my true Spirit has presented. **What is truly mine is this life to live: everything else is borrowed for the visit to Earth.** This is a deeply meaningful statement! The other thing to note is that the actual words carried meaning which was felt, or existed on a more refined level of communication.
    I then found myself in a large astral room which had fine furnishings. The most profound image was of two mirrors, very fine and flat, which were opposite each other and therefore the reflection in each was repeated into the deep distance within the mirrors. Iterative images are related to fractal geometry which is the nature of the Cosmos. Genetics is fractal code (for example every hair on one's head is not coded, but rather a fractal expression of hair which is changing with time exists). The 'reality' a human sees and the astral dreams we dream are a reflection of our ever changing being and this implies that reflections get reflected upon repeatedly. If you think about any of these words, you will likely think about what you thought, and think about it again. Contemplation is an iterative process.
    The next astral image was surreal, a silver mirror ball, with a backbone of silver metal, like a string to a balloon. Then the urge to send it off to the other realm because this Cosmos was not accepting it here. Since it is again mirror-like it relates to a thought bubble and the fact that we send our thoughts out to the aspect of the Cosmos referred

to as the past. Thoughts do not manifest as if magic spells, but they do have a lingering aspect and are stored in a numinous state. They are information and also influence intention. Sometimes they are forgotten completely and then surface again. Our body's neural network is a connection to the astral realm, which is more fluid and open than the physical Cosmos. The message of these poetic thoughts is that what one thinks does not disappear, but lodges itself in the past and the past has momentum pushing on the present (as well as the future pulling on the present); therefore, logically one should refine one's thoughts.

Next came an image of little people in green cloaks with hoods dancing and laughing. The message was, 'Why are you hiding this type of music?' I play a meditative flute and while being a listener of all different music, I felt this referred to some ancient tradition of multidimensional music. It seems that really deep musical secrets of sound are still hidden and although I seek to find them, I only find threads of them buried amid traditions that have been modernized. The message that followed was, "He gracefully and with great lucidity stepped away." Those who hold some ancient keys are still in hiding from those who would pervert and commercialize the power of the keys of magic music. Then the message, "All through the next morning the visions and meditations will continue." I understood morning to mean the time of the awakening of humanity to greater dimensional reality.

Next I perceived a relic, a golden box with two front doors holding a mystery. It was on the left side of what was happening (implying an artistic presentation rather than a logical one). I could feel it held a portal or a paranormal living force. It was locked away to prevent it from messing with our constructed reality. It was conveyed that it was not something evil, nor good, just a force to be reckoned with. The captors are afraid of the unknown, which may be wise but is more likely foolishly missing some great lesson or other benefit. This is a paradox which we all face when facing the unknown and which intensifies our consciousness. Should a door be opened and if so, which one or both?

The next message was, "A long obscure road lies ahead through forests and towns, not quite in the modern world (view), where old ways still prevail." As much as a murderous power group seeks to eliminate the wisdom keepers, they prevail and the messages are hidden in plain sight. The keys are presented in mythology which holds a deeper wisdom which few can comprehend. The message followed, "Beware of opening a portal to somewhere, because you don't know what might come into our world from the other side." So a paradox is presented which represents the state of modern humanity. We need to comprehend the ancient wisdom, but without the superstition, the cultural conditioning, which is baggage without value to a modern human. Many extremely intelligent humans explored Consciousness and had the advantage of slower lives which allowed vast resources of time and human energy to be dedicated. They were free of many of our conditioned myths of philosophical materialism which constrain the possibilities we would consider, while also making them prone to the mythological symbolism of personification.

The next astral dream message is, "After searching and having a cold case, a storm giant stomps down its foot and a footprint records its passing. **When a higher dimensional entity or phenomenon touches or passes through our three dimensional bubble, the dim reflection we perceive is elusively mysterious.**" A synchronicity has a very personal and intimate knowledge of one's being. Without personifying or humanizing the sentience, somehow the Cosmos operates in a mysterious manner and Consciousness is a primary factor. We can intend synchronicity. The final message of this meditation is "Are we able to be revealed in the light of a greater omniscient sentience and be OK without our sense of privacy?" Many ancient tales imply some humans lived in this light and the time will come, bidden or unbidden, when the presence will make itself known in our lives. This meditation invites you to be prepared, to be able to answer 'Yes'.

Session 0080:

SAUH: Out-Breath Sah, In-Breath Uwhhh with H fading to silence).

I contemplate giving or sharing energy with specific people, without recognition or seeking anything in return. A simple fact of my nature is that I am an energy generator which provides the energy (prana, chi) to others and thus they have their own being generate autonomous experiences. I am not influencing what they experience, I am just supporting a sacred space for the experiences to arise within them. I am not doing this with any egoic intent, but simply as my nature is to radiate.

The Mantra is the Heart mantra, implying the mantra of being loving and it is from a loving feeling that I radiate. This is the love for a baby, a child, a young person, a grown person, an elder. It is compassionate love which recalls the happiness and joy as experienced by children and allows the adults meditating to feel those flavors again; to recall in their own lives when being alive was vitality and bliss in action, in doing, and exploring. It is curiosity born of wonderment.

Then I entered astral awareness, but not through my 'third eye' on my forehead, but through the 'second eye' of my chest. This is much more primary than the refined third eye, as the astral fills the body and also radiates outward. The astral flows with the breath and has a sensual quality which imparts vitality to one's consciousness. Space seems very open and fluid and the presence of the Devi-s is felt without any image of them. There is just the divine loving presence offering grace and protection. It has the qualities of different beings, but is also felt as a unified supporting energy.

Then amid the swirling astral colored fluidity I saw my hands with the eyes in the center of my palms glowing with the white/clear light of the crown energy. I moved my physical hands to allow the flow of energy from my hands to surround and empower others non-locally. I also accept the meditating energy from around the world and transmute it, reflecting it in purified form. I do not know these people personally, but feel their good energy and feed them potential energy and let that living potential energy do its own work for them, providing them the experience which serves their highest good. In this way I am a servant of the Devi energy and not seeking, yet receiving insight as well, in that my Heart Eye is open and active.

Then at some point I find myself in an astral garden of light. It is beautiful with transcendental colors flowering, blooming quickly in fractalizing patterns of intricate ordered geometry. I linger there for a while. It is very sensual and yet more refined than sexual energy, but the Silver Cord of the second chakra which connects to the dreaming body is stimulated in a more clarified and purified energy. This resolved into my whole body being a radiant glowing node in the interconnected circle of meditation. **My Heart Eye was fully open and what is considered the aura, which is really infinite luminous superstrings of entwined relationships within greater consciousness, is sensed with the utmost delight.** Bliss is filling every aspect of my being as I offer others a share and receive from them a share of their energy.

Commentary 06:

I must comment here upon this cosmic language, so that it is not reinterpreted in terms which present a false picture of reality. I am seeking to describe what our language has no words for. The art of meditation, once one has cultivated it for many years, allows our consciousness to open doors of perception or sensory channels which are part of every human's birthright. But as in any art one pursues, much dedication and practice is required to be clear and proficient. What might initially be sensed as bliss in the body or floating in a heavenly sense of void must be experienced with ever more clear consciousness. Once one is aware of the finer points and the movement of the potentiating energy, then one may seek words from our language which seem cosmic, but are actually very human perceptions. Do not seek to mimic my descriptions in your experience, let the potentiating energy unwind within you and allow awareness of the sensations and experiences which are unique to you arise. They will be as unique as you are unique. I hope these words I share inspire you to meditate and experience for yourself the wonders available to every humble human.

Session 0081:

SAUH: Out-Breath Sah, In-Breath Uwhhh (with H fading to silence).

The Heart Center rests between the Base and Crown and nourishes both of them with every breath. In a sense it is like an infinity sign, with the crossing current at the Heart Center. The exhale corresponds to a rising channel of energy from the base to the crown, while the inhale sees a current of energy returning to the base and vitalizing the whole body. Soon it feels like my whole body is vibrating with energy. I sense that the energy is healing.

The Blue Devi's eyes are like black pools, the surface of which reflect me, while their depth presents a deep longing. They change and I see one eye and then both. They twinkle in brilliant colors. The changes reflect me and she seeks to attract me, to fascinate me, and to captivate my attention. Her eyes only appear as black mirrors due to my limited visual ability. When I see her truly, her eyes are the most spectacular eyes I have ever seen.

Then she causes thoughts to arise or I dream the teachings: I just know I am not in my waking thinking state and the phrases arise with clarity. The first is 'Intend Synchronicity', a teaching phrase from 'The Celestine Prophecy' and the second was, "Allow arising to pass through." The present experience can be viewed as changes passing through consciousness. Intending synchronicity is the process of increasing awareness of specific changes which are both statistically unlikely and also personally very profound. The complexity of all that we perceive as the ever-changing present is far beyond mental processing and we focus and pick elements to 'think about' from memory and even to be 'aware of' from conditioning. The phrases are complimentary because by releasing some of the mental analysis, which reflects on what has already passed through consciousness which is always present in the now and being in the current sensory flow, allows one to experience a more complete flow of the changes.

Then the phrase, "Must not the ego shell be broken for the chick to hatch?" The way it is phrased is as a question and the feeling that resulted was a reaction: I don't want to be broken down any more, I have suffered enough. But then there is the understanding that the ego is what suffers, not the real me. This is not an invocation of pain, but rather of freedom. It is the ego as a shell which traps one in conditioned responses and also limits one's awareness within experience. It is when the bird of consciousness flying through time is free, that it can truly explore and experiencing new wonders which it would have filtered out in the mental world view. **The ego personality becomes fluid and one's awareness increases to catch the synchronicity in the changes which are continually happening and offering one wisdom.** Then when the time of reflection comes, the thinking mind discriminates and determines the true synchronicity from the coincidence. While one might say, there are no coincidences, yet there are many correspondences of changes, events, situations, or occurrences which are interconnected which are not pointing out a wisdom teaching. The teaching is to be continually re-birthing, becoming new and renewed.

    Then I astrally perceive a blue circular ring holding within it a yellow core which permeates the blue circle and radiates. Every in-breath energy rises to the crown and every out-breath energy returns to the base of the body, the center of gravity, the first eye. In breathing there is the radiating flow which fills the body, the heart, and the crown and radiates through the three eyes all around a living being. It shines from us, but is a fluid like energetic substance of perception. It is continuously flowing as the bellows of the breath pumps life force. When it is powerful , its vibration is felt internally and externally. One's boundaries are permeable. One's shell of form is a container which is receiving energy and transmitting energy continually as vital life force. This energy is stunningly beautiful and shockingly powerful. Mental awareness of this vital fluidity which is itself consciousness as awareness is supremely glorious and yet remains the most subtle mystery.

Session 0082:

SAUH: Out-Breath Saaahhh, In-Breath Ooohhh (like moon, H fading to silence).

    I was very focused on breath, its powerful healing effect and also the connection to the atmosphere though the in-breath. My awareness was expanding beyond my boundaries and I was vibrating intensely. Then the words, "Not a Space Mic", floated through me. This implied that I could not hear the actual vibration of space, the song of the Cosmos. As a human it is important to accept limitations and even more accept one's current level of the power of perception. This returned me to my vibrating human form, not my body, but my astral body which assumes the same form, but is subtler. In this mode I saw the blue energy field with some red energy weaving through it, pulsing with every breath.

    The next words to flow through my mind were, "That means we have gone somewhere in life." Note that there were no intervening thoughts over the five minute time I estimate from the previous sentence, therefore there was not the mental process at work, but the more subtle astral dream flow. **If I interpret this statement it is saying that being able to focus exclusively on a mantra and use it to ride in the astral realm is one of the most rich journeys available in life.** Doing so in a drug free manner is an accomplishment in life which death cannot erase.

    At this point I perceive the left side of my conscious being to have an opening and I allow the astral field to slide around my perception until it is right before me. In waking life we would turn to look at the opening, but if the astral one is centered on the axis which is stillness, then everything moves about one's still locus. Before me the blue-red field seemed to have a vertical slit, a fold which the astral rushed into and out of. As I stood before the portal, I saw the Queen Devi and she had a bright point of white light on her forehead where the third eye would be on a human. It did not look like a physical feature, but rather a dynamic while light which she controlled and used both to perceive with and also to transmit her intent.

    Finally she faded and I was in a small A-frame cabin looking out the end which was all windows: a triangular wall of windows with several frames separating sections of it. This was brief as the meditation ended by circumstance, but I got the sense, the feeling, that this was a place to meditate and also to enjoy a natural view. One can create a personal sanctuary in the astral realm and return to it, but such spaces are temporary as are the physical body and all form.

Session 0083:

AUM Shakti Devi Hum: Out-Breath Ahhh, In-Breath oommm, Out-Breath Shahk, In-Breath Tee, Out-Breath Dev, In-Breath Vee, Out-Breath Hum, In-Breath Mmmm (fading to Silence).

The first impression was of a ball of many strings which signifies the superstrings of our being, the luminous strands of consciousness which make up the human form. We associate all sensory data as a complete world view, but the data has separate qualities and the simultaneity of these data flows allows us to find a cohesive world view, but they are each filtered in that we place different amounts of awareness on them depending on the situation. We almost never are aware of all the data we are receiving.

Then in the meditation I got the sense of how the different configuration of the luminous strings of consciousness in males and females results in very different world views. Men and women do not perceive the same data in a situation and although every person is different, some qualities can be generalized as differences. In a situation such as two couples going out to dinner, the male and female experience of the event vary differently. This goes beyond what the conversation was and has to do with the feel of the event.

Then I sensed the Cosmic Flow, the Power and Momentum of changes falling from the future and how it appears to be guided by a sentient plan. It does not honor our individual ego personalities, nor cater to our wants or even our perceived needs. **Situations appear to challenge us and to refine our being as consciousness.** We are carried through the changes of growing and aging bodies and the temporary journey shatters any static notions we might have. The river of time races along and no one can hold anything the same for very long, therefore as we breathe the mantra, we continue to have new and varied experiences. What arises can be teachings if we are willing to contemplate the experience.

Finally I was involved in contemplating that all our consumption, on every level, brings about transformation. We do not have a choice in the fact that our bodies require us to consume on many levels. Every biological entity transforms its environment and in an ecosystem the checks and balances between species makes for a very gradual and controlled transformation, such that all species involved are sustainable for ages. As humans have broken out of the natural constraints of our form, we have not yet gained the insightful wisdom required to be sustainable. **Earth changes brought about by our global transformation of natural systems will teach us that we are an integrated part of the Earth and the ways of the Earth are transcendental to our powers.**

Session 0084:

Aum Shakti Radha Hum: Out-Breath Ahh, In-Breath uMmmm, Out-Breath Rahd, In-Breath Haa, Out-Breath Hoom, In-Breath Mmmm fading to silence.

   Intuited message, "Let Shivaya put the lost souls into the oblivion of the past": I am to focus on my life, embrace my life and live to the fullest. Do not let anything stop me, share Tripping on Meditation. Then I sense a sweet smell within the astral space, which indicates the Devi is present. Knowing the sacred Devi is always present and yet experiencing the smell of paradise brings great peace.

   I am then looking down on a Wolf running in the forest. The Wolf is a noble creature. Wolves marry for life. They keep the environment healthy. Humans are predatory animals, but are not by default noble creatures. Some humans are much more dangerous and nasty than wolves, but some humans can be the supreme noble creatures who have compassionate love for all. Nobility is only supreme when an equal amount of humility balances a person. No one is greater or lesser, but a few awaken to their essence and are supremely noble.

   I then flash on music I used to listen to, which carried a spiritual message, but I do not listen to music with words very often anymore. At one point the endless words made me tired and I saw that the battles of intellectual ideas are foolishness: how do we live? I am thankful to the musicians who created the music of my youth, yet now I am inclined to instrumental music which allows me to meditate or contemplate the arising of my own thoughts and ideas which are in tune with the great song of the Cosmos.

   Radha: pleasure blessings of delight are offered. There are big cats surrounding her as her protectors. One needs courage to know the heavenly pleasure of the sacred Devi-s. The red inner and yellow outer astral space force fields merge into orange. Dark blue is still pulsing through it. My consciousness is both within me and without, in the Cosmos. A murmuration of white dots flies around the vast space and then groups into a triangle, I then find myself holding onto a gear, a piece of the machine connected by a rope like force field and playing tug of war, I assume with one of her cats. **There is no technology, nothing material which can do the work one must do to refine one's consciousness and commune with the Devi: only meditation which requires nothing more than breath and intent.**

Then I perceive white light forming a portal and it has a rim like a ripple and its ripple can open other portals. I see a huge tree, life's tree, and we are all within it. I see lines of people seeking, like bugs trying to get into the screen of a window, yet they each hold the key to realize they are integrated within the tree of life in their own spiritual hearts (Hum). It is just a change of perspective out of the mental and into being the consciousness which is aware of the mind. **We each have the door to freedom within.**

Session 0085:

Hari Radhe, Hari Radha, Radharani, Devi Devi: Out-Breath Rod, In-Breath Hey, Out-Breath Rod, In-Breath Haaa, Out-Breath Rod, In-Breath Haa, Out-Breath Rah, In-Breath Nee, Out-Breath Dev, In-Breath Vee, Out-Breath Dev, In-Breath Vee.

The first image was of the Blue energy forming a plus sign pattern and dividing the mostly yellow astral field into four quarters. Then I saw beautiful Devi faces, feminine blue Goddesses expressing supreme beauty. After they took turns looking at me and causing me bliss, they faded into the astral field. I then briefly saw a fox. The fox is clever and playful, they adapt to wilderness or a city, they are resilient and yet they keep mostly out of sight. It is a great blessing to glimpse a Deva's or a Devi's presence, even if the form mimics a human face cast in blue astral light.

I perceive a sheet of clear glass with white frosted patterns, similar to some shower enclosures, but the patterns are dancing fractals. The impression is that the sacred is veiled. Then a black hole forms a portal and ripples radiate out from it. I perceive fractal leaves blowing across the opening like a strong wind is present. Then I perceive the sacred body as luminous blue glowing skin, but I am so close that I do not perceive form, only the sacred radiance, the trillions of superstrings which form the Devi's aura.

This is followed by seeing a black panther on my left looking in toward the center. Black Panthers are protectors, extremely powerful and confident. They are invisible in the darkness and represent the supremacy of feminine energy in the Cosmos. Then I saw it morph into a Raccoon, and for me this meant the coming of the Way of the Divine and Sacred like a thief in the night, all powerful and revealing every aspect of every beings lives. **I receive the phrase, "The Truth shall be Revealed".**

The next message sounds like it comes from an old radio and it states, "The diversion of science". At the same time I hear a clicking sound like our old tube TV used to make, but even though I am astral dreaming, it sounds like it is external to me and comes from where that TV used to be before we got a flat screen. Then an image of wet light, glowing drops of rain, falling from above with spiraling motion and forming a protective circle around me. I come to understand that there is always a sexual component to enlightenment, the sacred and divine dance together into union. The Deva is all powerful and the unconquerable Warrior, but the Devi conquers even the Deva with her love. **Love is supreme.**

I am enclosed in a protective astral bubble. It is all around me, but is expanded in layers. Then I get the image of a house, a simple, yet modern and powerfully designed space. Thus, my consciousness is housed in a body, in a dwelling, and within the Earth's biosphere and that is protected by the solar system and the Sun carries it spinning through the Milky Way.

I contemplate that it is difficult to understand why we do some things, why we make some choices in life. We have gifts to offer to the natural Cosmos and to humanity. I see a necklace with a gold wire-like chain and a precious stone. It is slipped in an iridescent bag and that bag is slipped into a velvet bag. I see the Blue Devi's face bowed in thanks and in service. Although she is vastly more powerful than I can conceive and commands the Cosmos itself, she is humble. Although she is truly free, she is dedicated as a servant to bring enlightenment to us mortal humans bound in the flesh. Devi Hara Devi Hari (a next mantra is given).

I perceive a distant drum circle and a celebration of many diverse peoples dancing. The pain is growing upon this world. An upset voice informed me that there were mortals among humanity with intent to 'Punk You, Ron'. This means to discredit and rip me off of my energy and creativity. The message of this meditation is not to fear, but to stand firm in the sacred energy and open the doors by sharing the ultimate growth and healing power of Tripping with Meditation. It cannot be capitalized on, it is free to all. Chanting sacred vibrations harmonizes one's vibration and brings about resonance with divine astral states, a type of lucid dreaming while perfectly conscious and awake and aware.

One can look in the mirror of the astral and be revealed to refine their Way and become whole and at peace.

I then realize that every in-breath except the Ha of Radha run energy up the spine, the central channel, while Ha runs up the front of my body, up and in my senses. **As I follow the movement of the light of consciousness I realize that the science of sound is very advanced.** Something is not right upon Earth, since the ancients knew the power of sound and mantra, but the sacred wisdom has been suppressed. I then hear the astral reply, "It shall be revealed" and at that moment a crow caws outside the house where I am meditating.

At this point morning is calling and a large number of birds outside are chattering. I see that there have been so many lies told to me in my life and it makes me very sad. Who will be honest? Who will be transparent? Sometimes when my wife and I are sitting in the living room we hear sounds upstairs in the bedroom, but no one is there. I am alone in the house today meditating and I hear these sounds. I pay no mind, but our young dog, Rufus, who is about nine months old, and came from the animal shelter and from an abusive life, growls at the sounds and then barks and goes out to the porch and out the dog door to a small fenced dog yard while barking. I note this is the third external sound which was synchronous with this meditation. There is power in the words of this meditation. **There is a judgment day, a reckoning for humanity approaching like a thief in the night and the veil is thinning: every person shall be revealed, everyone will see and be seen.**

Session 0086:

Sri Hum: In-Breath Shree, Out-Breath Hoom.

I got the impression of a womb, being in the womb and my body holding my being, as well as the Cosmos as a womb. The entire creation as we know it, physical, mental, emotional, and astral bubbles circle around and holds our consciousness. I got the astral image of a mostly blue field, pulsing with scintillations of a red inner field of being crossed with a vertical and horizontal line, implying the four directions and a center, as well as sensing my own center of gravity.

Then due to world conditions and recent events of terrorism, I sensed the need to express compassionate love. **Violence and war are unacceptable behaviors.** They do not solve problems and in their conclusion everyone loses and there is great historic trauma which will carry into the future generations. Any belief, philosophy, or religion which advocates violence or war is a false doctrine and is having a negative impact on the evolution of humanity and the potential prosperity of future generations. Then my mantra changed:

S'ri Ram S'ri Ma S'ri Devi Ma Aum: In-Breath Shree, Out-Breath Rahm, In-Breath Shree, Out-Breath Ma, In-Breath Shree, Out-Breath Dev, In-Breath Ee, Out-Breath Ma, In-Breath silent, Out-Breath Ahh, In-Breath Ummmm into silence.

Just praying for the children in war torn places and those being traumatized amid all cultures. The children cannot conceive that the adults doing such things, only that they are monsters, and they grow up with fear and nightmares. Some live and suffer in war and others live in abject poverty and misery. Some live in affluent societies and yet are abused in many ways. Humanity is not civilized until every child is safe and in an environment that supports their healthy growth of body, mind, emotions, and intent. **Every child is a treasure which humanity has a duty toward.**

I then see a red point within a field of white energy as if a spear were piercing a field of pure energy. Children come to us with a lot of personality baggage, while having a purity of innocence about the world. When they are harmed by adults, their potential to contribute to humanity is harmed and all of humanity loses. Healing is possible and it is the duty of humanity to assist in global healing. Each individual must accept the trauma of their youth and in recognizing it and seeing it clearly, come to terms with it and heal to live as an expression their potential.

Sri Hum: In-Breath Shree, Out-Breath Hoom.

I returned to the mantra I started this long session with. I then perceived a hazy black creeping over the Earth: the biosphere itself is going dark as the light of life fades in species decline. This is a terrifying vision of the great extinction event now covering the entire planet and the cascading collapse is speeding up as I meditate. The image of a bowl, two knives, and one spoon. Soon there will not be enough food for the current human population. Science and technology are oriented toward war and with every war the biosphere suffers additional damage. Science and technology could easily feed everyone if that were where the intent was invested. The Earth's living and sacred body is being ripped to shreds by humanity's delusions.

I then saw three lines of energy and can only interpret that as the transforming of thought and language from a dualistic philosophy to a trinary philosophy. A trinary philosophy includes the circle of unity, while a dualistic world view propagates division, separation, comparing, and contrasting; rather than comparing and finding commonality amid diversity. A dualistic view is poverty and death, while a trinary view is rich and growing forever, fractalizing in ever new beauty. The three lines become the wings of an angel. Humanity needs a celestial being to come to our aid, as we are failing: failing the children and failing the Earth.

The final vision was of a ring of energy forming around the sun and a massive solar flare sending the energy of purification through the Earth. Imagining the Sun as an all seeing eye, how would humanity be judged? Yet I know many good spirited people, who seek to find ways to give gifts to humanity. For all the horrible acts of violence and war, there are more people who pray, envision, and intend for peace on Earth and good will amongst humanity.

Commentary 07:

This journal represents only my formal sitting in meditation. I often meditate without noting the details. I often wake up in the night, many times around three in the morning and lay in bed meditating. Sometimes I have powerful images. Occasionally the meditations slip into a form of lucid dreaming. This is different than being completely asleep in a dream and waking up, of becoming a conscious sentient being aware that I am dreaming, which very occasionally happens to me. This is like being in a full dreamlike state and yet riding on the mantra.

In one recent session I found myself in a room with soldiers, one in particular confronting a woman and her young daughter. I stood between the ill intent of the soldier and radiated at that lost soul that abominations are never acceptable under any condition and that no act of a living soul ever goes unseen or unrecorded in the subtle Akashic records, inscribed in the Plank level field of vibration. I held no judgment of the lost soul acting as a soldier, but condemned the actions which he was intent upon. I can only hope that somewhere on Earth a mother and her child were spared from the wickedness which is a spreading disease among humanity.

I advocate using mantra when going to sleep, when one awakens during the night, or as one wakes up for centering, but those sessions do not have the dedicated will and consistency of this set of experiments. Often at night or in ad hoc sessions my mantra shifts again and again since I have used many mantras for countless hours. It is this process of meditating at night, or sitting back in my recliner chair in the day, which orients me toward a specific mantra and provides the basis for these formal deep meditation trips which I am sharing in this journal. Sitting with mantra and slowing down the frequency of thoughts arising, one can know what is arising and perceive one's true reflection. Getting to know myself more truly and seeing the aspects which my ordinary daily personality ego ignores, I seek to avoid emphasizing results, successes, or cosmic experiences in a need for refinement of my humanity.

In meditation one gets to know their true self, which is neither the personality they present to the world, nor the personality which they mentally assume themselves to be. We all have many illusions and delusions to work through in order to come to the truth. **The truth of our naked being, naked on all levels, is a stark and awkward awakening.** Our assumption of internal invisibility and the privacy of our thoughts morphs over time until we are not seeing ourselves clearly. Our light of consciousness is directed by our spirit with focus and will to look at some parts of our nature and filter out others. **Meditation can help us see our own ego personality, not to destroy it, but to know it is a construct of this lifetime and to grow it consciously, refine it, and align it with noble purpose.**

I know there are times when the sense of someone abusing a child or torturing another human being, causes emotions to arise within me that if I had a sword, I would run the perpetrator through. I must be an old soul because my astral view is still visioning ancient weapons, rather than guns. I know that returning violence to the violent is not the solution and yet allowing the violent to continue perpetrating their sick ways upon others who are innocent is also unacceptable. Humanity needs a change of heart, where the feelings which dominate all our mental thoughts and belief systems are transformed in the wisdom that the Way is compassionate love.

The paradox of the Warriors Way is that the most loving and compassionate humans must sometimes take action against the lost perpetrators of horrors upon the innocent and undeserving. Every option at communication, understanding, and diplomacy must be refined and employed. **All of Earth's children must be protected and nurtured without discrimination.** The fierceness of the mother goddess should not be underestimated. The Earth will defend the biosphere through natural processes. As I write this it would be a lie to say that humanity is civilized! Humanity must realize that our ways need healing. A sustainable and spiritually rich future for all humans and the biosphere is possible. Let us together envision and intend with a strong will, dedication, and perseverance to offer the children of each succeeding generation nurturing which potentiates their utmost expression as contributing members to the whole.

Session 0087:

SAUH: In-Breath Sah, Out-Breath Ooh (as in Moon followed by subtle H sound) – flipping back and forth with: Out-Breath Sah, In-Breath Ooh (and in both cases the sound connects through the transition).

The first image was of a human physical heart, more of a graphic representation than a photographic image. This is the heart mantra and centers in the chest and represents love. Then I briefly saw the face of the Blue Devi and then it morphed into a bearded man, the Blue Deva, and I understood that these energies were powerful and could act as protectors. Then I felt a blast of energy from my Silver Cord which is the vast meta-entangled set of superstrings connecting my physical body to my astral body. I felt my physical body jerk in response.

Then the sense of acting as a disciple, as a student, learning from higher astral beings or from human teachers arose. It is not a matter of a teacher being higher or smarter than a disciple, but rather of having a specialized wisdom which the teacher can offer and share. Each one of us synthesizes all that we learn and if we are dedicated, we can offer the teacher gifts unique to our journey of wisdom in return.

Then the image of a trident was visible and I understood the paradox that the Trident can be seen as a weapon and at the same time represents the trinity of energies which make up the Cosmos. In a basic sense this refers to the continuum of form: time – energy/matter – space. In a deeper sense the trinity can be seen as the consciousness, the Cosmos of which it is conscious, and the experiential state of being conscious where the consciousness and the Cosmos are non-dual as an active process. The Trident as a weapon engaged in a battle between two forces is a dualistic concept, while the interaction, the drama of the story being written, is the real component occurring. It is through relationship that the Trident becomes symbolic. The image shifted to that of a Lion, not as a predator, but as a protector. A Lion as a symbol of power that stands firm with nobility demanding that the kingdom of humanity return to peace and that the innocent are safe and nurtured.

I then sensed the service work of carrying others over difficulties. Life contains sorrows and hardships, but together we can weather the storms much better than if we strive alone. I then had the sense of embracing a friend or loved one, followed by shaking hands with an associate. **In life our greatest treasure is to radiate with a heart of compassionate love.**

My next impression came of a great master acting as a disciple of a well-known teacher. The master was thus invisible and free to do higher work, while the well-known teacher was interacting with the public and therefore was bent by expectations. The heart seed mantra SAUH is about sending bliss, radiating with good vibes, and interceding in people's journey to being peace and some comfort in troubling times. There are many inevitabilities, not to say fate is fixed, but that there is momentum in specific matters. It is not given to mortals to know what is best, but rather to accept what is and help each other through the journey. The future will drop some surprises into the present. Together we visit the Earth to refine our compassionate love.

Session 0088:

SAUH: In-Breath Sah, Out-Breath Ooh (as in Moon followed by subtle H sound) – flipping back and forth with: Out-Breath Sah, In-Breath Ooh (and in both cases the sound connects through the transition).

The astral field was mostly blue and as I meditated I felt the swooning effect, where one's head droops and one is not very aware of anything except mantra which naturally follows breath. But refocusing a few times I perceived snow covered mountains. The vastness and the feeling gave me a certainty that these were the Himalaya Mountains. Once this was clear I was walking down a corridor within the stone of one of the mountains. It was a very ancient place.

I next perceived some subterranean rooms. There was a vast area underground, as well as a source of fresh water and also a pool of heated water due to closeness to geothermal warmth. In the rooms the walls were carved and especially in the water areas there were carved symbols and even statues carved from the rock. It seemed ages of humans knew this place and lived mostly underground, carving the stone and making every space sacred. They appeared to have intent to preserve some very ancient treasures of wisdom and also to transmit wisdom from generation to generation of wisdom keepers.

Session 0089:

Shri Ah: In-Breath Shree, Out-Breath Ahh.

Within the blue and red field I perceived various critters in symbolic form, and then the mature Queen Devi. I soon became focused on the five platonic solids and the many properties of quartz, reflecting on the old crystal radio design and the likelihood that many properties are not understood, since we are mostly aware in the limited, illusionary view of three material dimension of space.

Then again I perceived the Queen Devi and had a great longing to know her name, but even a name is a limited form and her beauty is deep and beyond all form. Human gurus arise and a few are true teachers, but Shri, a reference to the Supreme Devi, is the true Guru. A body is a temple holding a divine set of eternally bound superstrings through the effect of consciousness. A body is a sacred alter upon which the sacrificial fire of the eternally bound superstrings of a living spirit transforms the universal. **The totality of the Cosmos is the body of the Devi Shri.**

Then the outer yellow and green astral field were perceived with the yellow flowing from the astral sky through the green. My essence seeks a touch that which is real, an embrace from the Queen Devi that is intimate, not sexual, but that vibrates through my whole being at a higher frequency. It is a natural longing and it is neither good, nor bad, but a feature of being human. How can I be of service to the Queen Devi when she is so transcendental to my nature? How can I sacrifice my illusions to live in the Way as service to the unfolding of the divine and sacred Cosmos?

There is the tendency to seek to heal others, but I do not know what is in their best interest as they approach the door of death. **The human form is very humbling and a lifetime is a long corridor of life experiences which rush past the still consciousness, with the human spirit acting with intent, but subservient to the spirit of the Cosmos.** The body is the sacrificial fire and gets brighter as we grow and then dies down and fades, while some numinous essence is intensified and yet remains untouched and free. The touch of form penetrating deep and yet the core remaining fathomless.

Then I perceived tall trees in the inner red and blue astral field, surrounded by the green and yellow cosmic field. The opening was dimensionally above and the yellow streamed down into the green, as the blue fed into the red below. Our psychic powers trigger ego to assume one is powerful, but the Cosmos is the supreme power. Quartz Crystals are material and thereby limited to the receiving properties of their given form and even though we are vastly more complex, the human form likewise has well defined properties, limitations, as well as powers of reception and radiance.

As I continued to meditate my awareness was focused on my center of gravity (Hara, Dan Tien) in the pit of my stomach from which breath is potentiated. Being centered at the core one is vibrational and sensual. The life force is generated from the process of breathing from the belly and breath is a key to vibrant living. Then the Queen Devi appeared and indicated that her physical form is translucent, she is not as aware of materiality as we are. She functions at a very psychic level and her consciousness is radiant and entwined with many others who's forms are similarly translucent, not optically to physical light, but relative to the light of consciousness. I then perceived many strange humanoid beings who she works with and who are more similar to humans in terms of conscious evolution. The Queen Devi is dancing in the background of the movements of many life trees.

Session 0090:

Aum Kali Durga Hum: Out-Breath Ahh, In-Breath uMmmm, Out-Breath Kah, In-Breath Lee, Out-Breath Dur, In-Breath Gah, Out-Breath Hu, In-Breath Mmmm fading to silence.

The first thing I noticed was that within the dark blue red field there appeared thin lines of black filled with rainbow colors of every variety. They were to the left side and the bottom of my astral vision. Then one appeared right in the center vertically. They seemed like thin tubes of color that were rotating or that the colors were flowing through them in diagonal bands. They were just beautiful and that is the only impression they conveyed.

Then the message was, 'Taking the first one'. What this meant, I am not clear, but it is a societal tendency to lay more responsibility on a first child. Among siblings the youngest is often left to develop more independently of the parents control as the parents learn and also tire, while the first one often has micro-management by the parents. Durga kept bringing in children, their innocent and curious looks, but more mentally than astrally, more reminding about the grounded real care needed by children.

Then I saw an image of a Goddess, which seemed to change position and form. She appeared naked, but was only displayed in iridescent outlines, as if edges and boundaries were enhanced. There was nothing clear and around her was a room in a house or temple. She did not have any distinct features and yet she conveyed several feelings, as mother and protector. She was a warrior and yet was vulnerable in her openness and by being present. The complex multiple personalities were integrated and wholesome. She was focused on the children and the progression of generations.

The next set of feelings were of children abandoned by their parents, even while the parents provided a safe home, food, and other necessities; they were not giving the child (children) their time and attention, they were distracted by their own desires. They were not spending quality time from the perspective of the child's reality. They were more concerned with their personal desires. I understand needing to work and other aspects of modern life, but the Goddess was pointing out the truth of surrendering time and attention in interaction. Human touch is sacred and healing; but so is doing things together and communicating openly as equals in terms of the need for appropriate relationship.

Session 0091:

Aum Kali Kala Hum: Out-Breath Ahh, In-Breath uMmmm, Out-Breath Kah, In-Breath Lee, Out-Breath Kah, In-Breath Lah, Out-Breath Hu, In-Breath Mmmm fading to silence.

    Meditating on time itself, Kali being the feminine and Kala being the masculine forms. The first image was a tree of life, somewhat like a stylistic oak tree. An apt symbol, a living being with roots deep in the Earth and branches reaching to the sky. Then upon a red background I saw blue flower petals and in the center were green stamens with yellow balls of pollen. A flower's beauty lasts only a short while and attracts insects to help spread its pollen and form new seeds. I then saw a yellow background with some fractals of red, blue, and green. The background was large and the fractals small. Fractals are based upon a seed and an iterative process. **Life and genetic code is fractal in nature.** The Cosmos is a background for the fractal growth of Life.

    Next I was focusing on belly breathing and the cyclic nature of having awareness of the passage of time and then I felt myself rising as if floating upward. This was not bodily, but rather my consciousness. This produced a separation between my belly breathing and my point of view and then I had a new experience, a ring formed in front of my belly. This was visceral and I could sense it and it moved slightly to my left. It was about two centimeters long and had a diameter that I could fit a finger in, but I had no awareness of hands. It was metal and slightly cold. More like a piece of tubing than a ring to wear. Its solidity and my ability to sense it as an object outside of myself were unique in all of my memories. The startling nature of the sensation made it fade, as I wondered if I could control its movements with my mind.

    After a while as I settled back into breathing the mantra and was in astral dream space in a room and tried to put a large bowl on the right side of the upper shelf of a kitchen cabinet. There were already bowls there and I was unable to do it. Next I saw that the right was cleared out and was a yellow space, while the left side was in darkness. One must make mental space to receive new ideas. **A cluttered life does not allow the new to be introduced gracefully.**

Then I saw the globe of the Earth and then it was held in our hands, in the hands of humanity. Then I took the Earth globe and put it in my belly and began breathing through my connection to Earth. Then I saw a clear globe of crystal hovering in front of my heart and knew it meant to purify my heart space. It gradually became more transparent until it was invisible. In order to feel the environment one is in, natural or a human situation, one must be emotionally clear. To empathically sense someone's emotional state one must have a clear state in order to not project one's own emotions onto the other person and confuse what they are feeling with one's own emotions.

Then there was a diagram like a 'V' on its side and pointing to the left. It was centered and equal on both sides and had vertical lines segmenting aspects of it. Where the right side ended and it was open the lines became curves and twisted around each other. To the left was the point and the lines vertical became smaller and closer as the shape came to a point. It was a representation of two fields, the 'V' and the lines. To the left the space contracted into a complex microcosm and to the right it opened to a fluid macrocosm. **There are many scales to time which overlap as cycles within cycles.**

Then an image as if a bell curve vertically dividing my vision, the bell in the center extending from the right into the left. The right was yellow and green and the left was red and blue. The exterior world impresses itself into the interior world. I got the sense that what is required is a balancing and that our breath is the key through its cyclic nature. Our bilateral symmetry is only related to some aspects of our body and mind, while other aspects are to one side or the other, especially internally. Unifying the dual nature is empowerment: left and right, body and mind, functioning in a harmonious synchronistic manner is healthy and potentiates the optimum movement through the timeline of one's life.

Then images like drawings appear in various morphing forms: the Goddesses and Gods are sexual, like the tree of life, like flowers. They seemed to have a bizarre sense of humor as if to say that all personifications are an aspect of the onlooker, while the actor can intend a personality presentation, but it will be perceived differently by different onlookers. The Goddesses and Gods can adapt many forms, but in their essence they are formless. As one meditates, one realizes that they themselves are also formless and their form, while a precious vehicle for learning, continually changes and finally dissolves according to the bell curve of life.

Commentary 08:

At this point I have realized that the second syllable of the mantra most often ends in one of three sounds. Juxtaposing within the classic Tibetan Mantra one can align a great number of the sacred names as ending in 'I' (pronounced as a long E sound) or 'A' (pronounced as in 'Ahh') and the third ending of 'M' (Mmmm fading to silence and sometimes having an 'n' quality as it fades).

Note that thought sounds are not limited to the vocal possibilities of humans and the mind can produce sounds which cannot be uttered by the voice. Different languages include sounds which are difficult for a foreigner to learn. Likewise learning to make thought sounds outside of language, without reverting to onomatopoeia and just thinking of the sound abstractly is difficult. This also emphasizes that in meditation, one is not thinking of the sound, nor imagining the many attributes of a Goddess or God (which are themselves representative of a particular aspect of the one totality of divinity). One is trying to mentally vocalize the frequency and have that frequency resonate within one's core such that one knows intuitively, without thought process what the energy is conveying.

- Aum Mani Padma Hum
- Aum Hari Radha Hum
- Aum Hari Krishna Hum
- Aum Hari Rama Hum
- Aum Kali Kala Hum
- Aum Kali Durga Hum
- Aum Kali Krishna Hum
- Aum Kali Kula Hum
- Aum Devi Brahma Hum

- Aum Agni Soma Hum
- Aum Agni Svaha Hum
- Aum Shakti Shiva Hum
- Aum Sati Shiva Hum
- Aum Lakshmi Shiva Hum
- Aum Parvati Shiva Hum
- Aum Yoni Linga Hum

These are examples where the classic Tibetan mantra acts as a container and the second and third mantric seed sound displays this tendency. The vibration of these three specific sounds which can sustain and gradually fade into silence are a key feature of the keys to spiritual vibratory resonators which carry one's consciousness into specific wisdom spaces. There are particular internal sounds which can ride on the breath and bring one into a state of mind where one can be receptive to astral and intuitive wisdom.

As stated in the introduction, a mantra is not an affirmation phrase as the lost culture is teaching. Any sound cannot be a mantra and sacred sounds have a very powerful effect. Since the science of sound is so powerful and people are generally lazy or completely distracted by the external aspects of their life, the ancients used the names of the Goddesses and Gods to preserve the most powerful sound keys and then elaborate stories personified the various aspects of the Cosmic Consciousness.

Session 0092:

Aum Ambika Lalita Kalika Svaha: Out-Breath Ahh, In-Breath uMmmm, Out-Breath Am, In-Breath Bee, Out-Breath Kah, In-Breath Hhh to Silence, Out-Breath Lah, In-Breath Lee, Out-Breath Tah, In-Breath Hhh to Silence, Out-Breath Kah, In-Breath Lee, Out-Breath Kah, In-Breath Hhh to Silence,
Out-Breath Sva, In-Breath Hha fading to silence.

    The sound of these three Devi names are very similar and yet very unique. Again I think we can learn a great deal about sacred sounds by the vibrations traditionally used. I believe the ancients used sacred sounds as the names of the Goddess in order to preserve these vibratory patterns. The rhythmic pattern is also significant and while chanting the associations of first and second syllable or second and third gives different inflection: Ambi, Lali, Kali – Bika, Lita, Lika.
    A beetle like insect approaches me with a huge abdomen section. It is like a giant ball that it is dragging along. The feeling is that it is especially fecund and will soon lay a million eggs. This image was followed by an eclipse, which was a blue haze obscuring the sun, rather than the moon. This symbolizes a time of darkness upon the Earth, when things die from lack of sunlight. Then a brief scene of an Egyptian temple and it is known that a comet (or meteor) caused a global twenty year cold darkness (around 3,400 BCE) and this implies the history of Egypt rising from obscurity was a recovery from a dark time. Such events of dying impelled humanity's obsession with the unbridled desires of procreation.
    The next series of images began with a brief image of an explorer in a space suit or perhaps special work suit for underwater exploration. Then the entrance to a cave in a rock wall that had the design of a vulva. I am assuming we will one day discover many hidden places where records of humanity's past give birth to new understanding of our origin, whether in the civilizations underwater on the continental shelves or on the moon and mars. Then I saw three birds, but the one on the left soon was gone and then the one on the right was quickly gone as well, leaving the one in the center which started to grow. It was like a dove getting bigger and transforming into a white light.
    Then I saw a white face hiding behind a curtain of white fog and watching the drama unfold, remaining hidden while trying to uncover what is going on. This was followed by the symbol known as the flower of life and then other geometric mandala symbols in stained glass

windows. Some looked like cracked paint and others like spider webs, but all having a geometric nature. There was a lot of wisdom in the past which we could learn from, but time corrodes records and piecing together our long past will help us gain perspective on our current journey.

This was followed by a planet-like object crashing into the Sun and causing a great solar flare. In the solar flare I see a stream of letters, binary code, and symbolic words flowing out of the flare, seeking to leave behind a transmission, a message to be passed along after the destructive phase subsides. This is followed by morphing faces, modern and ancient, some intelligent and some fierce and angry, some like warriors and some like clowns, the whole gamut of strange human personalities vying to have presence. This implied in my feelings that what a human was is forever changed and continues to change. Finally the resolution was an image of a monk in a robe walking down a dirt road in a forest, carrying a staff.

While the patriarchy wants to write a male dominated history, and male creator, sustainer, and destroyer, the past honored the feminine energy and the channeling and nurturing of human life. There are many stories and aspects to any Goddess's name, but here is my impression. Ambika is the glorious compassionate mother, a fierce protector of the tree of life and also a sweet Goddess of love. Lalita is the Goddess of the play of life, the attractive one who leads the incarnate souls with desires, the director of the play of Love. Kalika is the time which washes away all material successes and informs us that only spiritual successes have meaning. These three Goddess control the three male Gods, the Creator, Sustainer, and Destroyer and remain transcendental. Therefore the Supreme Goddess is referred to as the primary Trinity, Tri-Devi, or triple Goddess. **One cannot understand the past by overlaying the present world view upon it, one cannot understand the present without seeing the past clearly, and one cannot make optimum choices for the future without clarity in one's understanding of both the past and the present.**

Session 0093:

Aum Bhairavi Parvati Sundari Shanti: Out-Breath Ahh, In-Breath uMmmm, Out-Breath Buy, In-Breath Rah, Out-Breath Vee, In-Breath Silence, Out-Breath Par, In-Breath Vah, Out-Breath Tee, In-Breath Silence, Out-Breath Sun, In-Breath Dar, Out-Breath Ree, In-Breath Silence, Out-Breath Shahn, In-Breath Tee.

Another set of Goddess mantras as the trinity of feminine power. The similarity in these three mantras is another clue to the nature of sacred vibration for enlightenment. In this case of using them with two breaths these mantras ground and center one in the bodies center of gravity, the Dan Tien, from which the power of breath originates. As such they are calming and healing.

The first image was of a dragonfly, which then morphed into a mechanical craft. This represented the Queen Devi as a sophisticated technological being. Then I saw the Blue Devi in a valley. The valley spirit is fertility and the spiritual heart where consciousness shines from. Then I saw a honey bee queen and her many devoted workers, a model of a hive mind or a neural network that has a main connecting power. In these images there is a centering axis which organizes the forces around it.

Then I descended into a memory of being at a club to listen to a band and a crazy American Indian man sat down at the table across from me. He was large and strong, talking of motorcycles and such. For most in the room he represented danger, but I conversed with him, even though I have no knowledge of bikes. My calm energy both attracted him and also stirred him up. He held great pain inflicted upon him for no other reason than being Native American. He was descending into rage, which was worrisome. Then a woman came up and sat down at the table. I added her to the conversation. He of course was compelled to flirt with her and she reciprocated. I of course slowly faded from their awareness and soon they left together. She was a rather small woman, physically powerless, and yet she easily led the powerful male. Gentleness and beauty are great strength. This gave me insight into the Blue Devi, frail and yet all attractive, beautiful and yet almost invisible. In her hiding was great power and by only revealing momentary glances of her glorious presence, my heart is enraptured. **What is our longing and how does it lead us on?**

Following this I perceived a green sunburst, a flowing outward within a blue field of astral energy. This is an apt image of the Earth's fertile growth over eons. It was followed by a vision of a beach resort in the fog. One would imagine going to a beach resort to be in the warm sun, but the fog has a mystical quality. It hides and reveals, making a place seem out of time or context, as if the resort could be from various centuries or could be located in many different locations. The Devi-s are mysterious and their hidden secrets are attractive. Their promise of bliss leads one toward their fierce and powerful nature which tames the great Deva-s, the most powerful beings in the Cosmos.

Then Radharani came to mind, the master of Consciousness personified, who takes Krishna by the hand and leads the most powerful one. Each of these Goddess is a reflection or aspect of the same power, the Supreme Devi. Our Consciousness is attracted by the external world and we are led forth and controlled by the sentient Cosmos, the dancing universe as a Goddess supreme. **The nature of time touching space and forming energy-matter is the triple nature which flows with an order within which Consciousness slowly awakens.**

Session 0094:

Aum Bharavi Sundari Parvati Uma: Out-Breath Ahh, In-Breath uMmmm, Out-Breath Buy, In-Breath Rah, Out-Breath Vee, In-Breath Silence, Out-Breath Sun, In-Breath Dar, Out-Breath Ree, In-Breath Silence, Out-Breath Par, In-Breath Vah, Out-Breath Tee, In-Breath Silence, Out-Breath Uumm (as in zoom), In-Breath Mah.

    I see a face and it sprouts peacock feathers with their mimicked eyes expanding like a fractal. Iterative systems reflect nature. Procreation is iterative and spawns more and more children in a divergent manner until some limit sorts through them. Repetition of mantra follows breath which must continue to cycle and each round causes the sounds of the thought words to vibrate more deeply and more richly, beyond sound that can be spoken.
    Then I hear a phrase, 'Go back and undo.'. While it is not possible for me to go back in time, I can revisit my doings and make adjustments to their current influences. I can return to a song I recorded and do a new version. I can create an art piece which is based on a previous piece, but holds a different message. The interpretation of memory and how stuck we are on recalling the memory and recycling the interpretation can be contemplated and one can release it to free the present. **One can change the path they are following if they are willing to commit the additional time and energy.** Sometimes a broken relationship can be mended, other times not, but in all cases one can forgive and release and face the future with a changed attitude.
    I open an astral door and enter a new floor, a new dimension of astral space. Information ripples. The concentric rings of thought meet other thoughts which change the pattern, and while the original inspired core idea-thought continues, it forms a more complex story with time. Again I find myself contemplating the iterative and fractal nature of our world view. **Everyone lives in their own bubble of reality.** The strands of reality are like drops of water on a spider web, interacting along supporting theories of the web, and yet individual and glimmering in the astral light.
    I perceive a golden temple across a lake from the perspective of standing in an open temple where there are columns slightly in front of me and to either side. One can idolize the other temple, but not being there, the perspective from a distance does not really define its qualities. **We perceive other people and their lives from a distance and imagine how it is or who they are, but we only get our personally**

colored perspective and everyone's inner perspective is complex and unknowable from outside of their life.

   The Queen Devi just watches, appearing neutral, and yet somehow curious or even fascinated. Why does a humble human like myself meditating attract such attention and why is it worthy of such attention. Even if I imagine that all vision is just dreams from my subconscious, why does a stable persona embodying superior consciousness watch. It is as if by turning consciousness around to contemplate its source with meditation that the Cosmos in some way looks back. Like a mirror looking into another mirror, the reflections reverberate and get finer and less detailed. The mantric vibration feeds itself and it feels as if the Queen Devi is fascinated by this continual process of my seeking out the deepest level of being which is beyond space and time.

   The trinity of the Goddess is unified and is one. It is our words which separate the Unity in order for us to understand. Time penetrates space and the boundary is the mass/energy form of the Cosmos flowing (descriptive words). The totality of the living sentience is far beyond these conceptual ideas. Words are symbols for ideas and ideas, like any reflection, have a much diminished dimensionality than what is. **Mantras are not words and using these vibratory keys to connect to the real transcends ideas, resonating one's Consciousness and entwining it with the Cosmos, the trinary Goddess, in a manner that is beyond words.**

Commentary 09:

If one considers UMA in ascending form (Starting with In-Breath uMmmm (um as in the oom of zoom), Out-Breath Ahh), it has the same letters as AUM in standard descending form (Out-Breath Ahh, In-Breath uMmmm). Therefore the difference is which transition is vocalized and which is silent. The syllables connect and therefore they roll together the vibration. UMA ascending resolves at the lower Dan Tien, one's center of gravity just below the navel from which breath originates: this is grounding and healing. AUM descending and then ascends ending up at the top of the head where breath ends: this is opening.

What is the difference between UMA descending and AUM ascending? The difference between using a mantra of these same sounds in the two ways is profound energetically. UMA has longing and intensifies one, pulling one into faster time. AUM settles one into being, releasing the push of the past to be now where time slows down. I am referring to real time as entwined with consciousness.

This also relates to Agni and Svaha. Agni as an in-breath puts one in the sacrifice of being in service to the Cosmos. Svaha as the descending breath takes one's sacrifice and manifests it as a life of co-creation. This as a very advanced meditational form where the top and bottom between breath phases are both open. This can be applied to the mantra just used (0094), but is beyond the scope of the present work. I am only mentioning it for those who have worked with mantra for many years and who understand how this is so.

Session 0095:

UMA: Out-Breath Uumm (as in zoom), In-Breath MAhhh -or- , In-Breath Uumm, Out-Breath MAhhh.

The first vision was of bed sheets, newly washed, smelling them, and feeling their texture: a very rich multi-sensory experiencing. What a pure delight to have a safe home and a bed. This is a privileged which many humans at this point in history do not have. It is a treasured feeling to get into bed tired and sleep. It is also amazing to smell and touch in an astral meditative state.

Then I saw a human woman and she stated that a politician was the worst type of human, indicating a specific politician, but this is not uncommon around the world. Very violent and selfish people push themselves up on the addictive adrenaline of power. Humanity would be far better off with humble leaders. Being a leader should be a service oriented endeavor.

Uma was a Goddess who was uncontrollably attracted to Shiva (who represents consciousness), but Shiva had a bad reputation as a naked ascetic. When one encounters the divine one is more than naked, one's inner world is revealed in the light. Then I contemplated the creation grounds. In modern society death is hidden away, feared, and fought against. Many people come to a terminal state completely unaware and surprised that death will come for them. I wondered about days gone by, how animals were dealt with. How some cultures held death as a sacred rite of passage. Humanity is slowly regaining knowledge that the dead, the ancestors, are not obliterated, but that their sentient core continues.

Then I saw Shiva as the lord of the dance (Natarāja), time being the consumer of all people and all their works. In my vision Shiva was red, like fire. The sacrifice that noble souls make, even accepting death if their service calls for it, is a supreme spiritual act. Consciousness dances within form, within the Cosmos, visiting Earth, but only for a short while. Living as consciousness and knowing the mortal form is rich beyond what a life in denial can offer is learned in meditation.

Finally I saw the Blue Devi's face and her right eye (to my left) flash in a green starburst which obscured her and then took on some tones of yellow. **The Cosmos is a coffin that consumes everything material, but we stop and dance in the now.** We can be aware we are consciousness and engage the Cosmos fully in a sacred and divine dance of life. Dance is being completely present in the movement of the Cosmos.

Commentary 10:

Since a lot of my meditation is informal, such as in bed either going to sleep, waking at 3 AM, or waking up in the morning and pausing before engaging the day, I am working with other similar sound Patterns.

- Ambika
- Amrita
- Lalita
- Kalika
- Krishna
- Bhairavi

In this case one can use 2 breaths as in Ambika: out-breath Am, in-breath Bee, out-breath Kah, in-breath silence. One can also use one breath which introduces a breath pattern, something I have worked extensively with for decades: in-breath AmmBee, out-breath Kah. Bhairavi could be a name with the Vee out-breath to compliment the Ah ending of the in-breath Buy-Rah or Buy as the out-breath (with powerful energy) and RahVee as the in-breath. There are also four syllable mantras: two syllable exhale and then two syllable inhale (three exhale and one inhale, one exhale and three inhale,).

- Sarasvati
- Radharani
- Bhagavati

Multiple syllables on a breath phase is advanced in that it actually involves a powerful transition from exhale to inhale and from inhale to exhale. These transitions are a type of pause and a thin place. **We perceive time differently when exhaling and when inhaling.** The two transition pauses are openings in the astral, portals like birth and death. One should use the single syllable per in-breath and out-breath for many years and explore the astral and its mirroring before opening these portals and experiencing the luminous total revealing of these portals. Being natural and balanced is the most beneficial path. **Do not proceed with ego, there is no goal in meditation although spontaneous benefits will arise in one's life.**

Session 0096:

Aum Kali Kala Hum: Out-Breath Ahh, In-Breath uMmmm, Out-Breath Kah, In-Breath Lee, Out-Breath Kah, In-Breath Lah, Out-Breath Hoom, In-Breath Mmmm fading to silence.

I am becoming comfortable with this mantra and the first image was of a scroll tied into a cylinder with a colorful cloth ribbon. While it could signify any sacred text, it felt like a diploma, as if some phase of this meditation process is completed.

I then saw a fox and it transformed into a possum and in both cases these critters tend to hide. Then I saw the back of a pickup truck with boards as a bed floor. It was well worn and yet in good shape. It was on a dirt track in a rural place. It seemed to have tools, a shovel and stuff. There was a sense of working and yet keeping a natural balance with the critters that live in the wilderness.

Then a transition into spoken words, audio as opposed to visual Hypnagogia. "The only thing is, archaeologists spend a lot of…" and the phrase was not completed as if to say 'time', 'energy', or some other well defined word combined to imply them all. I sense this implies they work on sites which satisfy their theories or sites which they believe they can write a paper about. The more exceptional sites and the oldest sites which are hard to fit into the current narrative are not explored, because the money spent must produce a viable paper and anomalous data gets rejected for many years. The current system of peer review can stifle science by trying to maintain beliefs rather than following data.

Anomalous archeological sites should be first to have their data published: without theories fitting them into the beliefs about how history was. There are two types of archeology; the data reporting and the theorizing of how things fir together, but these get joined to slow down progress in rewriting what we think we know. These should be separate data sets: the hard data and the theorizing about it.

"The deeper we go, the less we spend talking about this." Again a cryptic statement, but it is true that in these deeper states of meditation there are many feelings and impressions that cannot be quantified in words. This meditation contains feelings about deep time, Kali and Kala being feminine and masculine time, but I have very few words at my disposal. What does 'feminine and masculine time ' really mean? **Though I firmly believe that women and men do not experience or track time and memories in the same manner, I am at a loss to**

summarize this difference which could be an entire study of its own. The same goes for the most exotic archaeological sites, one gets feelings and impressions which have no place in a materialistic paper, yet intuition is a more advanced human ability than thought.

Then I see a heavy woman, not overly young or old, in a one piece tan robe who says, "I often cannot say it and I just have to…" at which point she puts her arms out with palms facing up. She radiates a warmth and attraction which is wholesome and accepting, as if to say she humbly accepts her state. Then I hear, "You really don't need to answer, I am happy in my birth". I find the word birth here to imply more than if she had said life, as it implies an incarnation and a visit to a specific point in Earth's space-time. A lot of personal memories which add up to a feeling about where and when we are born and our family. I sense she has a psychic knowing and though a mortal human with failings, yet has achieved a peace with her higher self's expression. The fact that she wears a robe, which could be opened, and yet isn't, provides another aspect to the feelings she radiates about the acceptance of her body and a lack of self-judgment, as well as a lack of desires. **Words cannot convey much that is felt in an astral vision and the unsayable aspects are the deepest teachings.** One can contemplate the image and statements and riff on possible meanings as I have, but there is an underlying organic experiential aspect to the feeling embodied in our memories.

Time is our memory and a most paradoxical subject to discuss. Music in the now is vibrations, but the song is formed through the memory which strings together intervals between notes. Our view of the present is shaded by memory and all we have learned to interpret over our lives. The past may be fixed and immutable, but our memory is not. We can recover buried memories of the past. Perhaps we are better off if some memories remain hidden or obscure. Siblings often remember events in vastly different ways since they have different angles of view. **The present is falling into the future and our ability to navigate is limited: in some ways we can control our destiny with dedicated intent and effort, but the future holds surprises and has its own designs.** This mantra is extremely powerful must be approached with great respect since it changes our relationship with time.

Session 0097:

Aum Krishna Radharani: Out-Breath Ahh, In-Breath uMmmm, Out-Breath Kree, In-Breath Shna, Out-Breath Rad, In-Breath Ha, Out-Breath Rahn, In-Breath Eee

I am inspired to add intent with my meditations and so I am indicating that I am changing into an next energy mode of clairvoyant viewing with the intent to both be present for other spiritual seekers and make energetic connection. I believe there are people around the Earth engaged in deep spiritual practice. I feel that some form of communication is possible and some type of sharing can happen which will benefit both parties. I do not seek to interject a change in their intent, nor to draw energy from them, but only to be present.

The next meditation also uses this, but then it also was explored in my private meditations. I do not hide these, but meditate a great deal without writing anything. It is important to me to spend greater amounts of time meditating, rather than writing, and also I have a life which requires activity. The peace of meditation gradually suffuses into one's life. There is an art to living daily life and ordinary human activity such as eating and working with lucid awareness, being present and fully sensually conscious. Taking time to read and contemplate many things is also valuable.

The first vision was as if a white pointer was making spirals in my vision. The I saw the Blue Deva's face: somber, peaceful, and observant. This was followed by the phrase, "I want to know what's going on with you?". This brought up a potential for a lot of contemplation about my current life. This was followed by the stripes of a tiger in the background, hidden in brush, and just glimpses of the color and the stripes of its presence. While I remain conscious that death lurks and hunts, I felt more like Durga, the protector spirit, was on the fringes of my consciousness as a guardian. **The astral realm must be ventured into with a pure heart.**

Then I intended clairvoyant viewing. I saw a couple in white robes hugging in a desert area. They were thin and willowy. They then just stood together looking into each other's eyes, perhaps communicating. In the open landscape and low hills that were quite distant there were occasional bushes, but the landscape was sparse. The environment was harsh, yet the couple were advanced spiritually and had love.

...

After a break (interruption) I returned to a deep state of mantric peace and continue in my meditation. I saw birds flying in the air and these were perhaps symbolic of spirits or the feelers of my spirit, the superstrings of connection that I was touching with my intention to find those doing the spiritual work for the benefit of the Earth.

The next scene was of a hall with a fire burning in a fire place. The place seemed to be stone or contain a lot of stone, like a temple or castle. Then there were people sitting in high backed wood chairs around a wooden table. The scene gave the impression of being modern, but having older furnishings. I could not distinguish the culture. The next scene was of people inside a large hall where there was a round stone cylinder holding a fire. The people were around the fire. I do not know if the first view where the fire place was seen at a distance was the same place, but there seemed to be a connection in the feel of the stone building. Perhaps this was a courtyard, because there must have been a way for smoke to ascend. One man at the head of the table was a big man with the features of someone who spent a great deal of time in the weather. He was both muscular and also had some extra weight on him. I could not distinguish features, but I felt he was someone carrying a burden.

Then I saw a man sitting before a low table covered in implements. Some of the objects were glowing, as if bottles or glasses with shining liquid and even solid objects with radiant light. Then I perceived an orange cross in a circle of white. This would be one of the oldest symbols, a sun cross, though later Christian iconography used orange in their crosses, this was equal length segments. It did seem like they widened at the end. Also it seemed there was some type of image over the large center. Then I saw a variation where instead of a white background there was a dark blue background. I am not inclined to search out what group might use such symbols because the groups I saw would not be on the internet.

Then I saw some pages of a book with big print and a lot of space between the lines. It had paintings on a few pages that looked like oil paintings. I could not tell if it was modern, a reproduction, or an ancient manuscript. This was followed by seeing someone using a candle to read on a low table. Then a vision of a big full moon.

The final impression was the phrase, "Waiting for The Time." I understood this to be related to a specific full moon. These images seemed to be a person or group involved in chemical magic, seeking to gain power through external means. Tripping with meditation is free of the requirement to use anything more than one's soul of consciousness. **There are no possession needed for spiritual work and the refinement of one's spirit.** If I am remote viewing a group, then perhaps my astral presence will inspire them to take the inner path of communion over the outer path of temporary gain.

Session 0098:

Aum Bhagavati Hum Aum Sarasvati Hum: Out-Breath Ahh, In-Breath uMmmm, Out-Breath Bha, In-Breath Gha, Out-Breath Vah, In-Breath Tee, Out-Breath Hoom, In-Breath Mmm fading to silence, Out-Breath Ahh, In-Breath uMmmm, Out-Breath Sar, In-Breath As, Out-Breath Vah, In-Breath Tee, Out-Breath Hoom, In-Breath Mmm fading to silence.

First I saw a young man teasing his mother about her friend and she was not complaining, but had peace with her doings. Then I saw a forest which then dissolved into a green astral light, which transformed to yellow, then blue, and then red. This indicates a path from without, being in the forest to within, being the consciousness dwelling in the individual body-mind ego. Then seeing a forest again I saw a woman in a red dress with a baby. The natural Cosmos is the mother of all beings and the ego wants to contradict the Way, wants to fight death, but nature just smiles and the Way continues.

Then I saw a Goddess which was insect-like, reminding me of a praying mantis. She was far more powerful that he Queen Devi, who although she is strange looking, is nevertheless humanoid. This was followed by a green cactus like rose which morphed into a red rose which finally resolved to a rose holding a center whirl of violet stamens with pollen. This is the same color projection from external to internal, but then the highest color, the soul of consciousness which observes the ego entity of our being, holds the seed mantra of creative power.

This was followed by a war scene and soldiers raping women and the terror of their children. The feeling of the trauma was palpable, conveying that it results in the children growing with hate and then into savage warriors seeking revenge. The Mantis Goddesses and Gods see the horror inflicted upon the children, the innocent descent adults, and the elderly and they detest the human beings who can perpetrate such heinous crimes. There is nothing unseen by the higher ruling powers and a complete account shall be reckoned upon these unconscionable soldiers and those who send them forth.

Then I saw a regal Goddess dressed in a green gown, with a golden headband crown with a large diamond shaped translucent green crystal over her forehead. She appeared in perfect human form. She was one who had born great suffering and yet stands noble and powerful. She is one who weighs all the deeds of humanity and will judge. No species continues forever and there are points in the evolution of many species when great purging occurs. **The feeling was that the judgment of humanity was approaching and the Earth Goddess would make a hard choice and cleanse humanity.** Meditate for mercy and live worthy of it.

Commentary 11:

I am at a crossroad in that several changes in my meditation have caused me to pause these long focused meditations and adapt my ongoing meditations in a less formal way. I often wake up around 3 AM and meditate in bed. I have no sense of time and sometimes I am meditating and hours go by, other times I realize my meditation is short and I fall back to sleep. I simply allow what is natural to occur. I sometimes meditate before afternoon naps, as well as at various times during the day. I sometimes meditate while playing shakuhachi flute. I am old and retired now, so I have the luxury of meditating more. I started working at age 14 and worked until full retirement age. Meditation has been a part of my life since I discovered it in tenth grade and has been a natural part of my life ever since. It has been healing and brought me a lot of inner peace from a very traumatic childhood and a hard life.

I have found a fondness for several mantras, and although I wonder about all the philosophizing stories around the Namah (the personified deity names). I most often just feel a resonance from the mental sound vibrations. A discussion of the related Goddesses and Gods is secondary to experiencing the energy which is extremely complex and beyond words. Each of us is a being beyond description, how much more so are the Goddesses and Gods.

- Aum Kali Kala Hum

  Meditations on time and the sentience which guides the unfolding of events.

- Aum Kali Kalika

  Attracting sweetness into the flow of my life's timeline.

- Om Hari Hara Hum

  A masculine form which balances and supports the above two mantras and attracts personal power.

- Aum Shakti Shakti Shakti

  - This Tridevi mantra is very calming and a great aid to falling asleep. But is also a mantra of great power to bring spiritual peace to Earth.

- Aum Shakti Shiva

  - This is a mantra of the Cosmos (Shakti) embracing Consciousness (Shiva).

- Aum Shakti Shanti

  - This is a mantra which is peaceful and relaxing, but has energizing power.

- Ambika Lalita Kalika: Sometimes in different order.

  - Trinity: Time + Energy/Matter/Form + Space; the essence of the totality unfolding.

- Agni Soma

  - A mantra for rejuvenation and healing.

- And others mentioned in the above commentaries of documented meditations.

There is another aspect which I embrace which is extremely powerful and energetic. It involves the point of change between the in-breath and out-breath. This is all I will reveal at this this point because it is a matter of awareness and involves all mantra work. It is an advanced teaching and one should follow the methodology presented here until it is mastered and then the more advanced method can be added and used.

Session 0099:

Om Bhagavati Devi Hum: Out-Breath Ohh, In-Breath Mmmm, Out-Breath Bha, In-Breath Gah, Out-Breath Vah, In-Breath Ti, Out-Breath Dev, In-Breath Vee, Out-Breath Hum, In-Breath Mmmm fading to silence

    First I perceived a yellow dome clearly amid the yellow and green pulsing astral light. This is a good representation that our external world is a sensory bubble. The mind extrapolates and combines the senses into an expanded world view, but our senses wrap around our consciousness like a bubble. I then saw something like a yellow head or a yellow craft flying around the bubble. This was a morphing image that represented another consciousness looking in. **Every living thing is in its own bubble of sensory data and although we share the quantum field of energy which is the Cosmos, it is our agreement on interpretation that makes it seem like we share the same world.**
    I then saw a yellow flower with an orange center flying up vertically. This was followed by an ice cream cone with orange ice cream also flying straight up. Orange is red and yellow and this represents that our inner world and outer world are inextricably linked. **Everything that we do which changes our inner state, also changes our sensory stream of data and therefore our world view.** This change is everything from the grossest sensations to the most refined perceptions being perceived differently. A flower smells good and is aesthetically pleasing, while ice cream tastes good. These things make us happy and our emotional state also changes our sensory bubble. **What we focus on is a key element to the world we view ourselves as living within.** The quantum flux of something called reality is unknowable and the subjective reality of a person and the agreed upon subjective reality of humanity are natural concocted world views of thin slices of what is.
    There is a feature of astral perception which is a shifting flow. The entire field will sometimes flow in three dimensional space, toward or away, left or right, up or down, spinning, or at any angle. It will often flow like a river in three dimensions and then shift fairly rapidly, but smoothly, to another direction of flow. I have no interpretation of meaning related to this phenomena at this time and the fact that it changes makes such interpretation difficult. This is an aspect of the astral realm which will require a detailed study. It must stabilize and become still for astral images to appear, therefore in meditation the goal

is to stabilize, which sometimes just requires patience for a natural settling that occurs when breathing a mantra.

Within the shifting field I started to perceive two metallic sheet, silvery gray, which finally resolved to be like curtains which opened to a view a stage in a vast amphitheater. My view was from above, not as a person on stage, and yet I was also observed. The observers watching the play were vast in number and their seats extended beyond my view. I got the impression that humanity is being observed and our drama, which we consider so personal and private, is not. This applies to every person's life, which is like an improvisational role in a play, as well as the collective actions of our species.

Then I saw faces, strange humanoid faces of all types. Of course some features reminded me vaguely of various animals and other Earthly life forms, but that is all my mind has to compare to. They each had a different character, a personality with a mood which gave the faces various demeanor, some fierce and some tranquil. None of the faces were threatening. They morphed rapidly and I felt I was being shown the vast diversity of nature. Devi is Maya Shakti, the supreme controller of the play of life, mother nature herself, which has blessed me with a human form to contemplate and see the play which I am entwined within. **All personification is a literary device for story telling: the Cosmos has sentient intent, but transcendental to personhood.**

This was followed by seeing a forest morphing into a savanna. This is a longer time scale where species emerge and species disappear. Life becomes ever more evolved, and when a species devolves or no longer fits the changing environment it is replaced. The amount and refinement of sensory information available to newly evolving species holding consciousness increases. Consciousness becomes more aware. In the Cosmos worlds are born, they evolve, and they perish. Every embodied consciousness is riding on the ever changing wave of the present. Meditation through awareness of mantra vibration with breath is the act of surfing that wave, riding on the edge of time.

Session 0100:

Soma Agni: Out-Breath Somah In-Breath Agnee.

After a pause of just doing personal meditations and not writing while meditating, but going deep without much focus on commentary, I have shifted modes and using two syllables from the most common mantras which I have a personal affinity toward. This was the first set I worked with. The first image was coals of fire glittering red within a blackness that the blue was merging into. Then the astral visual field started to cycle with my breath. As I breathed in Agni to the upper pause the field turned blue and as I exhaled Soma the field turned red. This was contrary to what my mind considered logical, but was repeatedly verified in the meditation. Then I saw little red, almost white, dots in the deep blue of the upper pause and blue, almost white, dots in the deep red of the lower pause. These became patterns like star constellations, but I could not recognize them.

Next I saw an abstract head of an old man, somehow I recognized that he was not from modern times. He was worn by the sun, powerful, stern, and yet a very wise teacher. Then the image morphed into a younger man who's eyes became white and crystalline, flickering with circular patterns. Humans are changing, but the new man was disempowered and his eyes no longer had the piercing consciousness which probes the mysteries, but rather just reflect light in a manner which had lost mystical vision. This I take as a warning for humanity.

Next I saw a red bowl holding blue liquid and then a blue bowl holding red liquid. This was followed by a funnel shaped vortex of blue in a red matrix. I realized that the ascension into the upper astral and the descent into the lower root of body consciousness were interconnected as if by a worm hole. **The Blue Devi appeared sad, as humans are mostly unaware of their inner quantum portal which fluctuates and gifts us with breath.** The colors shifted and the upper pause was green and the lower pause was yellow. The inner cycling matched the outer cycling.

I then saw a round face of a fish, smooth like a catfish, but very round with teeth and big black eyes. In myth spiritual dragons live the first part of their lives as a creature resembling a catfish. Teeth represent a gateway which protect the entry into the portal of life energy. This was replaced by a golden face of a person which became yellow, representing a refined person. **Next a serene vision of the Blue Devi's face, very beautiful and happy; followed by a sense of deep aquifers: there is no limit to the amount of living energy which is available to every person.**

Then I saw a city and temples built along a sacred river followed by a vague image of a crystal city in the sky. It felt like the river city and the crystal city were connected and both required the other. Our bodies and senses support our minds and astral selves and a fully integrated physical life potentiates a subtle meditative life, which together make a whole person. The Blue Devi smiles on the integration of all the levels of life, the visible and the invisible.

Next I saw yellow flowers on green stems. Then I saw mushrooms sprouting as the fruits that they are. In both cases the roots support the life in the world. Then I saw the Blue Devi with rich luscious red lips and knew this was her sense of humor, also the act of communicating with visual drama. **We humans are organic beings, our bodies and physical life in the world is as sacred as our astral visions.** The left side of my astral vision then became a yellow light, like a beacon and then the right upper field of vision became a blue radiance. The outer life we live is within us and the inner life we live radiates outward from us.

I then became very aware of my heart center and the Blue Devi appeared, but morphed into a red male face which appeared mad. Our bodies are often not happy with us. The Earth environment is not happy with humanity as a species. Then I saw the Blue Devi dancing and twirling in a cyclone of yellow light radiating from her heart. The whole vision of her spinning and the whirlwind then became white light, slowly becoming translucent and fading away. Our heart center is the key of balance. We radiate our feelings from our heart center. Mental wisdom is symbolic; only by feelings, by emotional vibrational state, may we choose to live our life with true wisdom.

A vertical opening of vibration appeared and an organic portal opened. I then got a message, 'A Celestial Being must be heart centered to radiate spiritual energy'. Then I got an astral blast of sliding energy which distracted me and I struggled to retrieve the message. Afterward a message came, 'Opening the spiritual Heart can be very painful'. This I understand, as the more in-tune one is psychically, the more one feels the vast suffering of humanity. The needs of the hungry world floods the telepathic web and the thunderous screams of the tortured souls within humanity blasts one's heart, yet one is called to radiate with loving presence and not succumb to withdrawal and reinstating numbness to the spiritual energies of connection.

Next the infinite energy of the inner worm hole portal was clarified. Energy cycling between the root and the sky, flowing from the heart along the back to over the head and down the front to the heart and down the back to the root and up the front to the heart. **This circuit is reflected in the infinity symbol and as the energy cycles, we breath.** The field breaths us and the open conduit draws in life force for rejuvenation and good health. The field is inherent in the Earth and the Cosmos. The two syllable mantra ascends from the core center at the bottom pause of breath, between the syllables at the heart, to the upper pause as Agni offers Soma, the waters of life, which descends to the heart between syllables and resolves at the lower pause continually cycling throughout our lives.

Then I saw a yellow dome in a green astral field and a yellow head-like craft flying above it from the left. This was followed by seeing a yellow flower with an orange center growing from a green stem. I sensed the flower was a healing herb. Then I saw a yellow ice cream cone with orange ice cream shooting up the center of my vision like a rocket. I took this to imply happiness of enjoying good things is also a healing balm. **Accept good things into a humble life and relish the beauty which nature provides.**

Finally there was great shifting in the astral field. This is like the entire three dimensional space around one's perception is moving dramatically. From the shifting emerged a reoccurring vision of giant metal doors which seemed to open like a curtain to a vast arena with seats ascending out of view occupied by all kinds of advanced beings watching the stage which was below and in front of my vision. I zoomed into the faces and they were all kinds of alien beings. I sensed the Earth is a stage and they are all watching. Are we ready to be aware of the vastness? Finally I saw forests shift to become savanna and this made me aware that many beings had been watching for ages as we evolved and will continue to watch, but now the show is in a period of intense climax.

Session 0101:

Agni Soma: Out-Breath Agnee, In-Breath Somah

    I reversed the syllables per breath compared to session 100. I again sensed red above and blue below. While above, such as my mind's eye was visionary, it seemed below was where space opened out in an obscure manner, but as a more dimensional and real space. Then I saw a green spiral, like a whirl toward a center point and then the green accumulated yellow and bound it, held it within the spiraling and carried it toward the center. The outer field spirals around the inner field which spins in response. The celestial cycles of the Earth rotating, the Moon phases, and the seasons turn within our bodies.

    Next I saw a vision of worker ants and then perceived how they were just part of the colony. They had lives, but were completely dependent on the organism of the hive. They had something like devotion which impelled them to accept their place and be of service to the whole. It was like the hive was their larger body, something they felt more intimately than humans feel their family or clan/cultural group. The hive was their higher self in a personal manner. The idea of a human being as an autonomous individual does not match our true nature as part of the biosystem and the society which supports us.

    Next I saw the Queen Devi as a child, with her big eyes curious and loving, innocent and vulnerable. She was precious and my emotions became parental, defensive, and of service. Next I saw her as taller than me, as if I was the child and she was big. I wanted to look her in the face, but she towered over me. **This provided insight into the nature of a child's perception, when adults are giants with vast power.** In this case the huge Devi still impelled a desire to look in her eyes without shyness or any shame about my limited being, because I was complete in myself.

    I next saw a vertical staff in the air and several cross bars of different lengths were at right angles crossing it, their centers joined with the vertical cylinder. They were gathered around the top, but some were rotated and pointing in different directions. It represented more of an antenna than a staff of royalty and seemed to symbolize many connections, many lines of communication. **The Queen Devi is a powerful being of the central command of many forces.** She then briefly showed her predatory nature, but not very graphically, just as a brief glimpse which implied she was a warrioress and huntress. The way she did it did not cause me fear or a sense that I was the prey. Actually I had to recognize that this is also my nature and a part of all intelligent organic beings.

Next I found myself meditating with Agni on the in-breath and Soma on the out-breath. I am convinced that this is the natural and correct order. Switching back and forth I noticed the shifting energy flow, as if a mixing, but either way, the main current of life energy flowed with the breath and with the breath to mantra association with Agni ascending and Soma descending the currents being affected were more subtle. I briefly replaced Agni with Devi, but returned to Agni for this session to have cohesion. I maintained the switch to Out-Breath Somah and In-Breath Agnee.

Next I was viewing mountain tops rising out of a vast sea or ocean of water which had a calmness to it, as if it were settled. I sensed cities under the sea, lost to human knowledge. When finally uncovered and revealed to the point of consensual belief, this is a mystery which will captivate the attention of humanity and heal our vanity in the disrespect we are showing to the Earth.

Next I saw a river flowing from the valley between two mountain peaks. I felt a sensual nature from the river bringing life giving waters and nurturing the lands below. Then the light dimmed and the mountains became black shapes and where they met a doorway opened and there was light inside the place that the door opened to. The light was pouring out of that open door and into the valley between the mountains. I sensed this was a teaching about Consciousness, the true light that lights the world which is our perceived reality. The river flowing was the light radiating and it was life's source pouring into the Cosmos.

Finally I saw a crystal landscape, a vast plain of crystal points which had a lavender to violet coloration. Upon it was a set of crystals that had a form. I tried to recognize it, but it was not complex landscape, a mountain, a city, or a machine. It had design and held some esoteric meaning in the construction of it. Then a hummingbird flew over the plane and this is a symbol of a spiritual messenger. Together these images indicated a good omen and not to worry, but to let time unfold as I follow my intuition and explore the Cosmos with meditation.

Session 0102:

Devi Soma: In-Breath DehVee, Out-Breath SoMah

    The first vision was of children and then of a baby and I understood that in these stages of life one has immense life energy flowing. The river of life flows through mothers and into children and birth is like a waterfall where a new vessel is formed for a ray of Consciousness. There is a moment after birth when a baby seems to intensely perceive its environment and then melts back into bliss and feeding. Children are popping with curiosity and learn at an incredible rate.

    Then I got the message to walk a little to allow emotions to settle: 'A little' meaning not a power walk to cover distance. Walking slowly with sensory presence to be completely present with the environment and without thoughts in order to settle into one's center is another form of meditation. This reflects the nature of children to move and act spontaneously. I remained seated with my eyes closed and simply noted that the practice of mindful walking is a complimentary practice to meditation. I also noted that even when shopping, one can be centered and present in the environment. Mantra meditation gets one out of their thinking mind, but also allows for a clear and sharp intellect.

    Then I was informed that: 'The Cosmos is the divine body and one should not stop at...' I take this to mean there is no mental knowledge which can contain all the secrets of the Cosmos and one should always have the wonder and curiosity of a child. Indeed, when my soul-spirit is continually amazed at the ever deeper depths of the Cosmos, then I can perceive and contemplate the source of life energy and vitality. The wisdom given was that I should not stop at answers in words, but that I should feel the answers in the pull of the cosmic design which is ever unfolding deeper mysteries.

    Fear damages the body, inhibits metabolism, and also limits one's freedom to make the choices which are the path of one's true nature. Life on Earth is a continual war of spirit. The depreciation of the feminine and the subjugation of women is leading to the failing of the human species and the collapse of the biosphere. **Humans have the illusion that ascending is attractive and grounding is undesirable, but only through being fully human and humble within one's natural life, will one experience the higher and more subtle aspects of life.** The higher vibrational sensory powers of the human form are manifest through the support of the clear awareness grounded in the here and now situations of one's life. A life of compassion and service is the way to awaken in deeper meditation. One cannot escape responsibility and achieve some imagined enlightenment. This is contrary to the popular lies people like to hear about reaching enlightenment according to some method or by taking a class. One's personal life is the class and the teaching are continuously falling from the future into one's life's path for refining the verb of living as compassionate love which is enlightenment.

The in-breath and ascension of energy is followed by the release and the descent of energy, the returning to the source, re-grounding every breath. It is with power that we breathe in and it is with surrender that we exhale. One must rest in order to have one's full vitality recharged to live with personal power. Getting must be accompanied with giving in order to be a beneficial process. There are things in life that we have a choice about and there are things that we must accept. Our bodies are the sacred art of the divine and must be respected in order to facilitate an astute mind and spiritual senses. Balanced living is healthy living: we are just visiting through our bodies and accepting our nature and caring for our personal body potentiates deep meditation and the insights which meditation brings.

Session 0103:

Hari Hara: In-Breath HaRee, Out-Breath HaRah

The first vision was of a snake face which I would interpret as a warning from a guardian and then it morphed into a primate, which looked very intelligent, but rugged as if living with the Earth. Then I was looking out of a cave entrance and there was a forest all around. The cave was above the forest floor in the side of a mountain or cliff. There was a blue sky. All together this is a statement about evolution. The teaching started with a glimpse of a snake, which was both a food and a danger to primitive man. I must note that Hara refers to Shiva, often pictured with a snake about his neck, while Hari refers to Vishnu, a warrior avatar, and together they represent two cosmic forces in harmony and coexistence of the unity of ultimate reality (Brahman). **Personification of cosmic forces as Gods and Goddesses, or as intellectual mental concepts, never implies that there is not a supreme unity to the totality of what is.**

Without elaborating long and involved wonderful stories, this is a power mantra, better for energizing before a contest or a test, than for sitting still and dropping into astral waters. It is extremely energizing and empowering. It insights rapid breathing easier than slow breathing. This is a warrior's mantra in this meditation's experience of it. All mantras are very versatile and have complex energy as celestial vibrations which invoke vibratory states in the meditating person, therefore one may also need power on various levels depending on one's current state of health and life situations.

Next I saw the inside of a cabin, which was well kept and neat, like a place that would be rented or was someone's getaway retreat place. I looked into the bedroom and a queen sized bed had an embroidered bedspread. The wooden walls had book shelves, there was an end table with a lamp and a small writing desk. Then I saw a sitting room with a chair. The walls seemed to curve and the layout or design was not clear. The rooms were small, but I did not see the whole place. I had the sense that it was in a remote location. It was familiar looking, but I can recall no memory of it. In meditation I wondered if it was a place I would one day visit. It was a strange follow up to the abstract beginning of the meditation being in a primitive cave dwelling. The images of the vision of it linger in my memory.

Session 0104:

Lalita Amrita: In-Breath Lahlee, Out-Breath Tah, In-Breath AmRee, Out-Breath Tah

    I was directed to focus forward, straight ahead, like traveling, and then I experienced the waves that breath me as expanding and collapsing. This is an important insight into the energy field that breathes me. Then I saw the Blue Devi, but her face was puffy and she had a red tear on her cheek. I sensed the wave breathing me as thickening and thinning. The Blue Devi's face turned yellow, but was still puffy. The gender became non-distinct. I understood this was theatrical drama. I theorize that the field shapes our human form. Her eyes then became small and beady like a humans: a reflection of how we are seen by the large eyed celestials. Her face then had a ghostly appearance, but very alive, just ephemeral as if from a realm with different dimensionality. I sensed nectar coming from my brain and down the back of my throat. Lalita is the playful one, the actress enjoying the fun of the drama, and Amrita is the nectar of immortality, the sacred nectar of life.
    Then I saw a guardian spirit wrap a coil of protection around my astral vision and the words, 'Does not want us to find him again.' This was followed by a vision of two small people. I do not know the meaning of these visions, but got the sense of being protected while exploring the sacred vibrations and their astral insights. The past has some periods of pain and suffering. Every choice humanity makes matters.
    Then I was in a very large empty room, like a warehouse facility, only empty. There was a massive window. This was followed by a theater like space and a group of people being briefed. Then I saw a woman sitting in a chair with a tapestry on the wall behind her, to my left. She looked like she could be doing a presentation with a feel of being comforting, like a podcast or TV interview. I felt there was a presence watching her, warning her not to speak about more than she was to reveal. Then I saw a fleeting vision of Yeshua (Jesus) psychically battling and winning against a reptilian demon. There was a sense of judgment and the woman's soul was being warned. She was in a dangerous place, but had to overcome fear to do the right thing and reveal the truth for the people.
    I returned to a bodily sense of my skin as a boundary, but it was vibrational and not a flat layer. The field was joining and parting, rising

and falling, thickening and thinning, and it was bathing my entire being and imparting a vibrational power. Breathing is like a bellows, filtering and refining the nectar of the etheric field, absorbing life energy and potentiating each living being. The key to long life and good health is natural deep breathing, synchronized with the higher dimensionality of the field which encompasses the dance of space and time which manifests where they touch creating the denser boundaries of energy and matter.

Session 0105:

Kali Kala: In-Breath Kahlee, Out-Breath Kahlah.

I find this mantra to be very natural and in balance with my life. The mystery of time is one of the deepest that a human can ponder. I first perceived a face with two colors, which then settled into a happy Blue Devi face. Her form was the opposite of austere, with a hint of plumpness in her dark skin. This was followed by ascending stairs, which I took to indicate the ascending way, which includes descending. It is the way of balance where discipline and dedication are accompanied by happiness and laughter.

I then saw a compass rose with a 'H' below where 'South' is traditionally and sensed that this was Hydrogen, the simplest and earliest atom. It represented the foundation and then I saw cyclic transformations symbolically represented. Everything grows from the most basic foundation and increases in complexity. Eons of generations of stars evolved into more complex stars as the available elements increased. Life evolves, terraforming the Earth for successive waves of more perceptive beings.

Next I was outside of a window. There were flowers in the flowerbeds. The window was wooden with frames of glass, like in an old house. One can see that the symbolism matches my age and my sense of windows which are not plastic or steel. I could see a person inside, but the image was vague. I understood this had to do with the conscious self being outside of the house where the personality self lives. My life is inside the house, but my soul of perception, my essence consciousness, is transcendent and looking in when I am meditating. Outside of the window, outside of the house of time, is the foundational nature, the ordering impulse. **Rather than consciousness like a star shining from the body into the world, the body and world hover in all pervasive consciousness.**

Then the idea came, 'that is all we see of others'! No matter how well we know a person, we are looking in and only have a vague sense of their inner person. We often overlay a person with our ideas about them and some may be close reflections, but many are our own reflection. When we approach a person with inner silence, and listen with our feelings, we can get a better sense of them. People close to us still have a part of themselves that is a stranger to us. None of us show ourselves completely openly, without filters and assessing how others would feel about spontaneous true being. Indeed, there are things that arise within ourselves, which do not represent our true nature due to continual bombardment by a perverse and demented programmed media which infiltrates many aspects of all cultures on Earth as a predatory parasite seeking to drain our power.

Next I saw a rainbow field of light. My whole astral screen was like a two dimensional curtain of scintillating rainbow colors. This was followed by occasional white shooting stars streak down from above. Then I saw a thick forehead and dark eyes looking into my astral field. I had the sense that I was being watched. **The astral realms are not an empty place.** What we consider as serious in our lives is just a game to the higher dimensional selves which we are, yet every choice we make matters. There is an astral presence mocking, but it has the intention of showing the foolishness of our ego selves, while it is also enjoying the absurdity of the play of who we think we are in time's stream. We have so many layers to our complex personalities which time will wash away. I then saw a stone and I saw cracks forming in it, even the solid rock does not endure times erasure.

I often have meditated with this mantra late at night and usually what remains is just a clearer mind, but once some words came to me: **"Enjoy the journey. Everything takes Time. Time Takes Everything. Enjoy the journey…"**

Session 0106:

Taom Mandu Hum HonSees: Out-Breath Taom, In-Breath Mmmmm Out-Breath Man, In-Breath do, Out-Breath Hum, In-Breath Hon, Out-Breath Sees, In-Breath silence.

This is a mantra which I developed as a personal mantra fifty years ago, but which I altered for this meditation because I follow what the natural tendency is, as the Spirit moves me. Taom is a combination of Tao and Om, Mandu I chose for the feel of the vibration and now I see that in Sanskrit it means Pleased, Joyous, and Cheerful. Hum is the Heart mantra of compassionate love. And Hon-Sees acts to ward off danger and harmful energies. Sees shows an emphasis that is like sheesh without the 'h'(s). The Way of the Word (Om, Aum, essence of consciousness) is Joyous with Heart centered Compassionate Love and wards off all contrary energies.

I first saw a mug, as for a warm beverage, with a picture on the wall behind it. The mug represents comforting goodness in life. Then the picture was clarified as a black with white stylized tree that had an aesthetic beauty of form. This morphed into other trees and then showing patterns of bamboo leaves. The final image was still a black background with the image in white of a bird, but as if the bird were formed of clouds or pure smoke. In summary this message is stating that aesthetic art has the nurturing satisfaction of a warm steaming beverage on a cool morning. Art feeds one's being with a richness that satisfies and brings a cheerfulness and joyousness to one's life.

While simultaneously being filled with beauty, the telepathic web is filled with people being tortured. My childhood was filled with abuse. Then an image of a red wall with yellow on it as if sprayed and having blotches without distinct edges and there was a window in it. Then I saw a wooden coffin against the wall and then the wall was the whole view. In life the duality of joy and suffering rises and falls like waves. This phase of humanity is a time of ignorance where suffering is the prevailing energy on the telepathic web. We are all connected and yet we are only responsible for the energy we send out. No one is responsible for the totality of humanity and yet every aware person feels responsible to do whatever is possible to bring healing. I then saw a little tender flower and had the awareness that it survived a vast powerful storm.

I then saw a symbol for vibration and know that all is vibration. It then formed an image of a sword as a symbol for freedom and yet the sword was oscillating, as opposed to being solid. Our vibrations, the energies we radiate in our feelings, thoughts, and actions are the sword of freedom. The vibration changed from the warding energy keeping the torture at bay (HonSees) to the heart energy and compassionate love which can overpower the suffering (Hum). We live in a time when the art of healing is being reawakened and the wisdom that all children, adults, and elders are equally valuable for the future of humanity, as well as awareness that everyone is entwined within human civilization. Love our enemies, but if a dangerous bear threatens innocent people, put it in chains. Love our enemies, but be warriors standing for the innocent and defending freedom. **The opportunity for every child to grow up with what is required to offer their gifts to the whole is the path to human prosperity.**

Session 0107:

Kali Krishna: Out-Breath Kah, In-Breath Lee, Out-Breath Kree, In-Breath Shnah.

Kali is Goddess of time, which erodes and destroys all form, but also divine feminine energy which protects the birth and growth of new life from destructive forces and nurtures the river of life. Likewise Krishna is a God who is a warrior that stands against the armies of those who aspire from the point of view of greed and who setting personal ego above the evolution of humanity. Both personifications, Goddess and God, are for telling literary tales, but represent the highest nature of the Cosmos which is beyond the reach of words.

The first image was ice in a bag melting and this can easily be interpreted after the meditation to represent the condition of the Earth and how the natural systems held the polar ice as if in a bag, or within boundaries, but now this system is broken and the ice is melting. This was followed by a tree lined driveway to a modest mansion. Two rows of trees were matched with two rows of bushes and the driveway between them leading to a house with two stories which was big enough for more than one family and yet was obviously just owned by a rich family and consumed much more energy than needed for a good and humble life. It is a reflection of societal imbalance and the abusive use of resources which is fueling the catastrophic melting of the ice caps. The dark Goddess and dark God warn of impending collapse of a system of life which is out of balance. My personal comment is that there is much hope for the future potential of humanity, but the meditation shows there is a problem facing humanity.

Next I saw the Sun as a phoenix with wings of yellow and red flames rising and encircling in a dazzling display of glory and then exploding. This then resolved into a blue sky with many clouds. The blue was rich and the clouds were white. Then I saw the Earth globe with its blue waters and its cloak of white clouds, but not much green, just brown land. While meditating this did not feel like a prophesy, yet reflecting on it we can see that the Sun itself could change life on Earth in response to humanity destroying the protective layers which shield us from the Sun's power. Kali's fierce form terrifies all mortal beings and Krishna's universal form completely overwhelms all mortals. **There are cosmic forces which control human destiny in ways we cannot comprehend and we must trust that the Cosmos which brought forth Consciousness through the human form over ages of time will bring a new phase where we can thrive.**

Then I saw a thick tree trunk followed by a huge green top of leaves: a very healthy and robust tree, like a mature oak. This was followed by a yellow ball of light streaming out in all directions and morphing into green fractal patterns. The sun fills the Earth and together they support the tree of life. The tree has a hardy trunk and can withstand many storms. This represents for me the continual promise of fecundity, that the Cosmos itself wills rivers of life to rush forth in the time stream. The energies of the Goddess, the essence of the living Cosmos as manifest, ordered progression holds the intent for life and receives the God energies of Consciousness arising within it; Consciousness perceiving the Cosmos ever more deeply and gaining ever increasing awareness is the twin duality and in their sacred union is represented the unfathomable totality.

Then I perceived the total blackness of the void and within it a blueish sheen arose and then it divided to a darkness to the left and a dark violet on the right and there formed a boundary between the two shades which danced in fluctuation. Then, on each side of the boundary, two red dots appeared and the boundary on the left seemed to wrap around the two red spheres, but this meant that the boundary on the right's center moved into the lefts area, maintaining equilibrium between the two sides. **There is a higher dimensional nature to the Cosmos and our three dimensional view is a very diminished reflection.** If one takes a picture of someone or themselves, it is a two dimensional image of a very complex being with a detailed inner life of many layers. In the same way our three dimensional view of the Cosmos is lacking dimensions which are currently unseen and unfathomable to us.

The many aspects of the divine feminine energy of time and change combined with the divine masculine energies of space and form can only be represented in word symbols in a very limited and diminished way, but can be experienced. The thousand names of Kali and the universal form of Krishna are far beyond the minds ability to comprehend and yet these transcendental aspects are inherent in human experience if one meditates deeply.

Session 0108:

Aum Shanti Shanti Shanti

Consciousness, the true Light that lights the Cosmos, and the Tridevi Goddess, the Supreme Sentience embodied as the Trinity of the Cosmos: the totality of Time, energy/mass/form, and space. The Word and Peace, Peace, Peace. This is the last meditation in this first experiment of documenting my personal meditations. I did not write more than short key notes while meditating. I usually do not write in my ongoing lifelong meditation practice. There is a spontaneity in my regular practice and the sessions I have written about here are very focused.

This meditation began with seeing creatures which were strange and bizarre, such as a long smoothed skinned being with a long snout and big human like lips. Then this morphed into other creatures and then into the Wild Blue Devi, and her eyes were dark with warning. Following this I saw a huge blue circle within a red matrix. Of course each color contained some of the other and the border was fizzing with the exchange, just like a person's inner and outer worlds continually interact with vibrant power.

Then I saw people all around the world meditating or doing spiritual practice which put them in communion. They were of all races, women and men, with different world views and yet communing with the one divine. Among them were ordinary people of the secular modern world, indigenous people, and people of different meditation schools. Some were alone and others were in groups. They were all acting for the common good of humanity.

Then my view shifted. **Be warned, the loudest voices within the human telepathic web are people crying out in great suffering.** Then I saw a woman tied up in bondage ropes unable to fight, being cast to the ground and her glasses broken. Then I saw blood as she was murdered and then I saw a crazed man who could not live with himself, but was terrified of death, hoping it was obliteration, but somewhere deep within knowing he would face his Karma. The telepathic web is filled with subconscious horror!

Then I felt the masses of innocent people in war torn lands, their lives devastated by the games of lost power hungry fools who think they are above the laws of karma, but death does not honor riches, nor mortal power. The suffering of children wounded and the suffering of parents losing children or other loved ones reverberates in the telepathic web. Then I saw the tools of the war lords and also the paradox of the true warriors defending freedom and standing up against the tyrannical dictators. I know peace does not come from violence and I also know the Warriors Way and the duty to protect freedom and protect the innocent. The cosmic dance of the Cosmos includes a predatory element and the paradox is that the Goddess as a divine lover and a nurturing mother, is also the supreme fierce warrior defending the sacred tree of life.

Conclusions:

The visual content of the meditation is primarily emphasized here, since it is the aspect easy to write about and the mind loves content, but there are many deeper aspects to meditation which have greater value, but which have a numinous quality that defy being symbolically represented in words. Initially the peace, calm, and bliss of meditation can seep into the body and one becomes healthier. There are a great number of scientific studies which prove this is true. This is augmented by internal mental peace which facilitates emotional balance and clear thinking. Neuroplasticity is the brain's ability to change and adapt throughout life. It's a result of learning and experience and is greatly enhanced through mantra meditation.

A dedicated meditation practice eventually leads to a person having a wholeness of being, a self-assured confidence, and a general high functionality in daily life. Meditation provides an avenue to heal from personal trauma and also creates an inner state to potentiate physical healing. Meditation is a powerful tool which teaches discipline over the mind and thus allows the mind to function with controlled focus on tasks, which makes one more functional in daily life. Meditation empowers one with the abilities to make their life journey a powerful gift to humanity.

Every mentally sound person should seek the vast insight available through mantra, but I must warn that not only that which is hidden within your being will become known to you, but also what is in the shared telepathic web of humanity and all of life. It is therefore critical that those who take this path are prepared for rapid change and growth. One will gain a more powerful presence and this will affect all of one's relationships. One will see through personal misconceptions (which is the normal process of personal growth) faster than one could without meditation. One will change at a quicker rate than before meditating.

It has been shown that when many people in a city meditate, the general crime rates go down. Meditation is one of the greatest forms of service to humanity. By reconnecting one's life with the spiritual aspects of one's being, one becomes a more functional part of humanity. By becoming more centered and increasing one's awareness, one will function in daily life with increased personal power. Mantra is an ancient art, but I hope that this work stimulates a new renaissance of meditation, supplemented by scientific inquiry which has already shown the vast personal benefits of meditation, but has not thus far yet documented the transformative power available to humanity through mantra.

Meditation is a mirror that allows one to know their inner self in greater detail and therefore to refine their outer journey. This can be difficult for those with a great deal of emotional and mental baggage and it may take years of dedicated practice to become clear inside, which allows one's true self to radiate out through their life's doings. Meditation allows the creative potential of each individual to connect to the greater whole of humanity and to refine all of one's relationships. Meditation is a powerful tool for bringing peace and taking humanity into a prosperous future. I believe Mantra Meditation is the most advanced form of meditation which one can use in this age. Let us all together envision a wonderful and joyous future for humanity and dream, play, and work together toward achieving it.

*   *   *   *   *

Each person is an amazing set of vibrations, cycles within cycles, harmonizing to allow one to be alive. Each Phenome affects the body, mind, and emotions in a very specific way. Mantras and phenomes were described poetically as having personalities, being Goddesses and Gods, because they are so powerful and have specific vibrations which can cause one's own vibrations to harmonize and lead to a healthier life. I humbly present this record of my experiential research and hope that Humanity embraces meditation in daily life for a healthy and prosperous future.

www.ingramcontent.com/pod-product-compliance
Lightning Source LLC
LaVergne TN
LVHW051825080426
835512LV00018B/2730